Healthy Eating Weight Loss Value Bundle

Zero Sugar Diet + Mediterranean Diet for Beginners

The Complete Box Set for Healthy Living

By Christina J Evans

Table of Contents

Just for You

A free gift to our readers

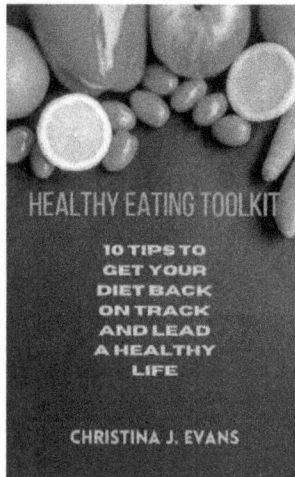

Click here

http://christinajevans.com/healthy-eating.pdf

Joining the HL Community

Looking to build your healthy eating lifestyle? If so, then check out the Healthy Living (HL) Community here:

www.facebook.com/groups/1004091000384321/

Healthy Eating for Healthy Living

A complete guide to zero sugar diet for beginners

By Christina J Evans

Introduction

t was a normal Friday. At least I thought so. My youngest daughter, Evie, had a bake sale at school so I was up to my arms in cookie dough and muffin batter the previous day. I have to say I was happy with the results. So much so, that I didn't mind sampling 'a few'.

The following day, I brought my daughter to school, and just when we were about to enter, she turned around, reached for the bag of baked goodies, looked up to me, and said "It's ok mommy. You don't have to go with me." I was surprised but I let her go, thinking she was probably trying to be a 'big girl'.

At the end of the school day, I was outside waiting for her when one of the other moms came up to me and said "Hey, you feeling better now?" Seeing my confused look, she said, "Evie said you were not feeling well and asked one of the other moms to help her with the bake sale." Somehow, I managed a "Yes, I feel better now" - just at the exact time I was feeling worse.

When I tucked my little girl that night I asked her as casually as I can "Why didn't you want mommy to help you out today?"

She looked at me and said "I don't like it when the other kids call you the 'black tent lady'. You know, because you only wear big, black clothes all the time." Oh. "And you probably couldn't help anyway." Oh? "We had to go set up outside and do A LOT of stuff and the other mommies are faster moving around, and going up and down the stairs. You're too fat to do that." And then she turned around and pretended to sleep.

And just like that – my heart broke into a thousand pieces.

That was the turning point for me.

FOR YOU – I'm sure you've had your own turning point as well.

- It can be seeing yourself in a photo and then suddenly being shocked at how 'big' you've become.
- It can be that judgmental look that complete strangers give you as they stare at your size. (It's worse when they do that at the grocery store or while you're dining in a restaurant.)

- It can be a friend, colleague, or family member 'innocently' making fun of your weight.
- It can be people always asking if you're pregnant.
- It can be the saleslady telling you that you should really try the dress you're holding in a bigger size.
- Worse still... depression may be hitting you or a serious health issue has come up that's completely negatively impacting your way of life. (You may even think – what life?)

I know all this because **I've been in your shoes**. In fact, ALL of the items above happened to me at one point or the other.

I wish I could tell you that from my turning point, all the excess pounds dropped easily and we lived happily ever after. But that was not the case. **I failed so many times.**

Over the next three (3) years, I would lose weight, gain weight... lose weight, gain weight... In the end, **I had put on MORE weight than when I started**. It was a very mentally draining and emotionally exhausting time. Every time I gained the weight back **I would sink into depression.**

The depression got so bad that at one point, **I started to become physically ill**. I would have panic attacks while driving, blinding migraines that prevented sleep, and during one beach vacation – yes, I was wearing something big and black to cover up myself again – **I had a heart attack**. My doctor said that I either had to be on medication for the rest of my life or lose weight.

By this time, I just wanted to throw my hands in the air. The only thing that stopped me from completely giving up was this – **I couldn't find the words to tell my daughter 'yes, mommy's a failure'**.

So for the nth time, **I tried again.**

And **THIS time, everything fell into place. I lost the weight - and successfully kept it off - for 10 years now.** And I couldn't be happier with my life!

- Imagine waking up wide-eyed, alert, and full of energy.
- Think of all the health issues – shortness of breath, all-day tiredness, heart problems, diabetes, joint pain, high cholesterol, etc. – that can be REVERSED.

- Visualize cutting your food budget by almost 50%(!) not by eating less, but by eating right.
- Look years younger as you see your hair, skin and overall appearance dramatically improve.
- Wear anything you want! Picture a wardrobe that's not 'all black and baggy' but made up of various styles, cuts, and colors you can wear confidently.

And perhaps best of all – imagine looking in the mirror and loving who and what you see.

Now, I don't think there's a woman alive out there who doesn't want at least one of the things I listed above, so let me tell you exactly what's going to happen.

I'm going to hold your hand and give you my step-by-step tested blueprint on how to cut sugar from your life so that you can quickly and successfully lose weight, and not gain a single pound back.

You see, I know what you're going through because believe me, **I've been there.** I've gone through so many 'fad diets' that I almost completely wrecked my health and my body.

So, when I opened my eyes and understood that **we were being fed LIE after LIE after LIE about how to lose weight**, uncovering the TRUTH became my goal.

Instead of just believing in whatever an 'overnight guru' was talking about, I buried myself in RESEARCH. Science became my friend. Licensed doctors specializing in female weight loss became my allies. This is why through the next pages you will see me frequently refer to published data and studies. **There is no hype here. Just truths.**

When I had collected enough knowledge, I created a **zero sugar weight loss plan** for myself. And I am not kidding when I tell you that **the pounds just started to melt away**.

All the hardship, all the illness, all the heartaches, all the disappointments – they disappeared as my excess weight melted away.

Soon enough, EVERY SINGLE PERSON I came into contact with would remark about my amazing transformation. Some would just ask how I did it, but many more would beg me to create a zero sugar weight loss plan for them too!

And I could never say no. How can I when I've been living under the shadow of obesity too for many years? And when you start to uncover what works, you always say to yourself – *if only someone told me the right way to successfully lose weight and keep it off.*

Well then, **let me be that SOMEONE.**

If you're ready to drop the weight and change your life – **turn the page** and keep reading.

To your healthy living,

Christina J. Evans
Female Body Fat Expert | Healthy Living Advocate

Chapter 1
Healthy Eating Guidelines

Q
UALITY OF LIFE. Many ebooks on healthy eating focus on weight loss and looking good. There is, of course, absolutely nothing wrong with the physical or aesthetic consequences of eating healthy. However, you should also keep in mind that with healthy eating you also achieve BETTER QUALITY OF LIFE.

Think about **living WITHOUT suffering from health- and weight-related diseases** such as diabetes, coronary heart disease, high cholesterol, high blood pressure, and so on.

Think about the **MENTAL AND EMOTIONAL STABILITY** that you will achieve if you NOURISH your body with good, quality food rather than just 'filling it'.

WHAT is Healthy Eating?
Healthy eating is eating REAL FOOD. It is ensuring that you are feeding your body with nutritious food and drinks to help it function at its best. It also means following a healthy eating pattern and consuming the right amount of healthy calories for your body.

WHY Should You Eat Healthily?
There are so many reasons to live a healthy life. And here are some of those reasons.

➤ Improve HEART health.
    Did you know that **heart disease is the primary cause of death for adults in the US?**[1] That sounds a bit grim but here's the good news – up to 80% of premature heart disease and stroke occurrences are preventable IF you adopt a healthy living lifestyle!

    A zero sugar diet automatically helps to lower blood pressure and keep your heart healthy. So you're on the right track.

➤ Lower your cancer risk.
    Eating healthy, good-quality food items means you're also eating food rich in antioxidants, substances that can prevent or slow damage to cells caused by free radicals. This in turn reduces your chance of contracting serious illnesses such as cancer.

Some studies have also found that a diet high in fruits lowered the risk of upper gastrointestinal tract cancers.

➢   Improve GUT health.

Our bodies serve as a host to a myriad of bacteria. This is a fact. The key is to keep a healthy balance between good and bad bacteria. If bad bacteria start to thrive in our bodies, our immune system weakens making it vulnerable to various diseases.

A diet low in fiber and high in sugar and fat promotes the growth of harmful bacteria. So, switching to a zero sugar diet is definitely beneficial for your gut health.

➢   Strengthen your bones and teeth.

One of the things that people don't realize is that by NOT eating healthy food, your body loses out on much-needed nutrients. For instance, calcium and magnesium are important for strong bones and teeth. You simply cannot squeeze these nutrients out of a *hotdog*.

➢   Improve brain function.

Research shows that certain nutrients and foods improve brain function and protect against cognitive decline and dementia. A low carbohydrate, zero sugar diet rich in vitamins, omega-3 fatty acids, flavonoids and polyphenols, and fish were in particular seen as great for improving brain health.

➢   Sleep better.

Do you sleep well? It sounds like an easy enough question, but did you know that 62% of adults around the world claim that they don't sleep as well as they would like.[2] If you don't get good quality sleep, instead of feeling rejuvenated the next day, you feel sleepy, foggy, and groggy. And this leads to bad eating choices, which in turn can lead to weight gain. How?

Some studies have shown that sleep deprivation lowers *leptin* (the hormone that tells your brain you're full) and increases *ghrelin* (the hormone that tells your brain you're hungry).[3]

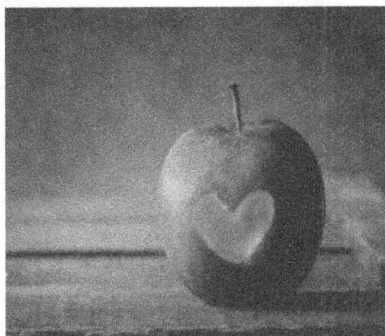

So, what you should keep in mind here is that one completely affects the other. If you don't sleep well, it's highly possible you'll eat more and make bad eating choices the next day (weight gain). But if you DO eat well, you increase your chances of sleeping well. So win-win!

➢ BE HAPPY.

We are what we eat. Studies show a direct link between what we eat and our mood. In fact, a 2016 study discovered that a **diet with a high glycemic load may cause symptoms of depression and fatigue.**[4]

NOTE:

You've probably heard of the glycemic index (GI). This indicates how fast 50g of carbs in a particular food item raises our blood glucose levels.

The glycemic load (GL), on the other hand, considers GI values <u>and</u> the total amount of carbohydrates in a standard food serving. As such, it indicates a food item's glycemic and insulin response.

See also <u>Appendix A</u> for a list of common grocery items and their glycemic load.

In another study, it was learned that a diet rich in vitamins and minerals is linked to a lower risk for mental health disorders including anxiety, depression, and attention-deficit hyperactivity disorder (ADHD).[5]

And let's face it - success at any endeavor makes one happy! Doing a zero sugar diet and succeeding at your weight and health goals are all excellent reasons to be happy.

➢ LOSE WEIGHT!

Excess weight increases your risk for chronic diseases. Luckily, a healthy eating lifestyle automatically promotes weight loss!

By simply focusing on the RIGHT FOOD to eat, you inevitably lower your calorie consumption. So if you're

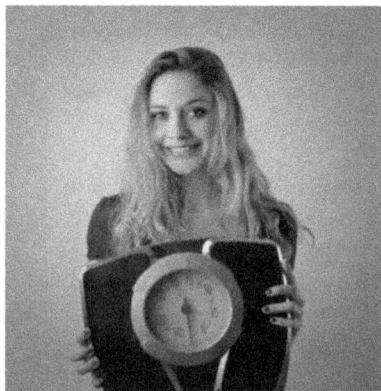

worried about 'calorie counting', don't be.

Eat well and eat right, and dropping the pounds will follow.

7 Tips to Increase Your Chances of Healthy Eating Success

In Chapter 7, you'll get a detailed zero sugar diet plan. But to give you the best chance of success, I suggest that you first do the following so that you're in the RIGHT ENVIRONMENT to succeed with your healthy eating, healthy living plan.

1. **Start SLOW.**

   Change is difficult. Many people who want to change their eating lifestyles do so with the best intentions. However, taking on too much too soon is detrimental to success.

   Think of it this way – **success builds on success**.

   You may start slow, but as the days progress you will notice small changes. For example, you may start to notice that you breathe easier, or that you have a bit more energy in the mornings, you may even start to notice some weight loss. Take each achievement and build upon it.

   On the other hand, if you make too many life changes at once, you may not be able to keep up with all of them. Things may begin to feel too difficult, making you give up and stop any progress.

2. **Switch to smaller plates.**

   Did you know that a bigger plate can make you eat more?[6] This is because our eyes like to see a full plate – no matter what its size. The great thing about switching to smaller plates is that you trick your brain and your stomach to eat less without even noticing!

   If you don't want to switch to smaller plates completely then switch what you PUT on your plates. For example, put healthier food items on your normal-sized plate, and less healthy ones on a smaller plate.

3. **Keep a food journal.**

   Many dieters underestimate the power of keeping a food journal. In one study, it was found that people who kept a food diary six days a week lost about twice as much weight![7] Here are some of the reasons why keeping a food diary works.

- **You become mindful of WHAT you eat.**

  Mindless eating or distracted eating is when a person is completely unaware of what or how much food (and drink!) he or she is consuming. This is why so many dieters THINK they're eating less, but in reality, they're not eating less at all. In fact, they may be eating MORE. Why? Many people who go on a weight loss program overestimate the energy they burn and underestimate the calories they consume.

  However, if you keep a food journal then you know exactly WHAT you've eaten and HOW MUCH you've consumed. But this is only half the equation. Once you have this knowledge then *healthy adjustments* need to kick in.

  For example, say you noticed you eat two (2) chocolate chip cookies every afternoon with your coffee. The average chocolate chip cookie contains approximately 200 calories. So now you know you consume 400 calories every afternoon just on two cookies!

  Healthy adjustment #1 -> consume only one cookie for a week
  Healthy adjustment #2 -> consume a different, healthier cookie for a week
  Healthy adjustment #3 -> substitute fruit for the cookie

  Your 'healthy adjustments' are all up to you. The most important thing is that you apply them. If you can, go 'cold turkey' and simply eliminate eating cookies with your mid-afternoon coffee. The most important thing is this: make a change that supports your new healthy eating ways.

- **You can keep track of any food allergies, issues, and sensitivities.**

  Keeping a food diary also helps you narrow down which food items may be causing problems such as headaches, bloating, indigestion, and others. For instance, she never really noticed it but after keeping a food journal a friend of mine noticed that chips (her weekend indulgence), and broccoli (one of her favorite healthy foods) were causing her bloating and flatulence! You can imagine how fast she got rid of those food items on her diet.

- **You can uncover unhealthy food triggers.**

  Are you a stress eater? An emotional eater? A habitual eater?

  Stress eaters, as the name suggests, are those who eat when they feel anxious or pressured. An emotional eater usually uses food to comfort themselves such as when feeling lonely, depressed, or bored. A habitual eater is someone who eats simply out of routine. For instance, many people tend to bring out the 'munchies' when watching TV after dinner. You're not necessarily hungry; you're just used to eating something while in front of the TV.

Discover your trigger for unhealthy eating, and you'll find a way to 'de-activate' your eating response.

For example, a friend of mine noticed that one of her food triggers is when she dropped off her son at her ex-husband's place for the weekend. She would come back home and start looking for things to eat. (Her food journal showed a long list of food items every other Friday night.)

So, to STOP this eating response, she started planning activities after dropping her son off. She visited a local swimming club and has been swimming every Friday night since then.

How to start a food journal.

A lot of people don't start a food journal because they overthink it! So just start. Don't worry about fancy pens, notebooks, and paper. Grab anything you can use. Although you can also just use your mobile device, writing them down is better.

Also, keeping a food diary is a habit you need to develop. So don't be discouraged if you fail to log something or skip a day or two. Focus instead on trying to develop a routine. Log items (what you eat AND drink) as soon as they pass your lips.

Log how you feel too after consuming something. For instance, after a specific meal or food item, do you feel good or stuffed? Energetic or sluggish? Take note and adjust accordingly.

BE HONEST. No one else is going to benefit from your food journal except you. So, there's no point in fibbing the details. By knowing and accepting what you've done, only then can you make positive changes.

4. **Acquire a support system.**

When embarking on a weight loss program, you may want to start 'quietly'. However, having a support system can dramatically increase your chances of long-term weight loss success. And I'm not just talking about friends and family members. Of course, if they support you, great! But your weight loss support system can come from other corners too.

Look around you. Do you have friends or colleagues interested in losing weight too? If so, talk to these people. Perhaps you can find a co-worker with whom you can have 'walk dates' after lunch or a friend with whom you can plan healthy cooking weekends.

Join your local gym. It's already filled with people concerned about healthy living, so you just might find your new fitness buddy there.

Consider online weight loss groups or forums too. There are A LOT of online groups dedicated to healthy eating and healthy living, and perhaps you'll find the support and help you need there.

You are making a huge, positive life change right now. And you don't need to do it alone.

Look around. Don't be scared. Ask for help.

You just might be surprised at how much your circle can GROW by simply reaching out.

5. **Minimize distractions.**
Often, life gets in the way of weight loss plans. You know how it is. A friend calls for a lunch date at a restaurant with too many high-sugar, high-calorie choices. Work deadlines mean working late (again?) and so you're 'forced' to order in food. There are many ways your best-laid healthy eating plans can be sabotaged.

However, you know all of this already, which means you can plan ahead and be ready for such distractions. Here are some tips.

- **Meal prep during the weekend.** You know that there will be times when you simply don't have enough time to cook a healthy meal. Fine. You know this. Accept it. Now, what are you going to do about it? You meal prep. Make a shortlist of quick and healthy meals you can cook or prep over the weekend, portion these out, and put them in your freezer. This way, you'll have a ready supply of healthy meals within arm's reach.

And don't think healthy meals are bland or boring! Are chicken nuggets boring?!? (Click here for healthy, REAL Chicken Nuggets recipe.)

- **STOP checking your mobile phone and/or computer first thing in the morning.** Focus first on having a HEALTHY breakfast, and perhaps even getting a short workout done in the morning before you put your mind on work mode.

- **Learn to say NO.** Saying no to someone or something is not being mean or selfish. It's simply you loving and prioritizing enough to focus on your health and fitness. Remember, you're supposed to live YOUR life, not someone else's. So do things that benefit YOU.

6. **Think of NON-FOOD related rewards.**
An eating lifestyle high in sugar conditions the brain to seek food as a reward. So before you embark on your zero sugar diet, have a go-to list of non-food related rewards.

For example, instead of a 'cheat day', reward yourself with a 'spa day' when you reach a certain weight milestone.

Here are other non-food related ideas to treat yourself.

1) Go for a new haircut.
2) Buy a new dress.
3) Buy/read a book.
4) Schedule a Netflix 'marathon'.
5) Book a massage.
6) Drive somewhere.
7) Book a facial.
8) Call someone and schedule an impromptu dinner or movie date (or both!).
9) Purchase a cooking gadget or utensil that supports your new zero sugar, low carbohydrate lifestyle (e.g., juicer, steamer, etc.)
10) Get new sports clothes/gear.
11) Take a day off.
12) Buy yourself some flowers.

7.   **KEEP AN OPEN MIND!**

Lastly, and perhaps the best tip of all – keep an open mind. Don't limit yourself. Don't disregard something just because it's new or you're not used to it.

In fact, many people new to the healthy eating for healthy living movement never thought they would end up loving something they've never tried before such as meal prepping or even cooking in general.

Remember, just because you've never tried it before, doesn't mean you can't or won't like it.

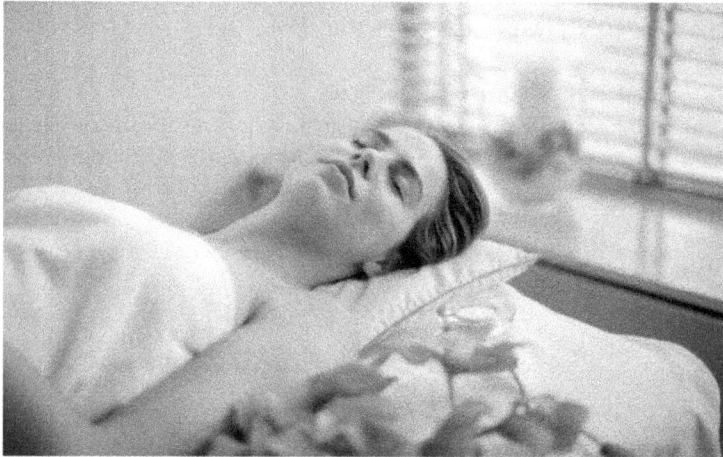

Chapter 2
The ZERO SUGAR Diet and How It Works

What's Wrong with Sugar?

Sugar is naturally present in small quantities in vegetables, fruits, grains, and dairy. Eating whole foods that contain **NATURAL SUGAR** is okay because, in addition to sugar, real food is also high in fiber, essential minerals, antioxidants, protein, calcium, and a host of other good things that your body needs to function well.

And since our bodies digest real food slowly, the naturally occurring sugar in them provides a steady flow of energy into our bodies' cells. (No sugar rush!)

The problem starts when we eat too much **ADDED SUGAR**. This is the sugar that food **manufacturers add to their products to boost flavor, texture, and extend shelf life.**

Keep in mind that **ADDED SUGARS do not provide any nutritional value or benefit whatsoever**. What do they add? **EMPTY CALORIES**, which lead to weight gain and illness.

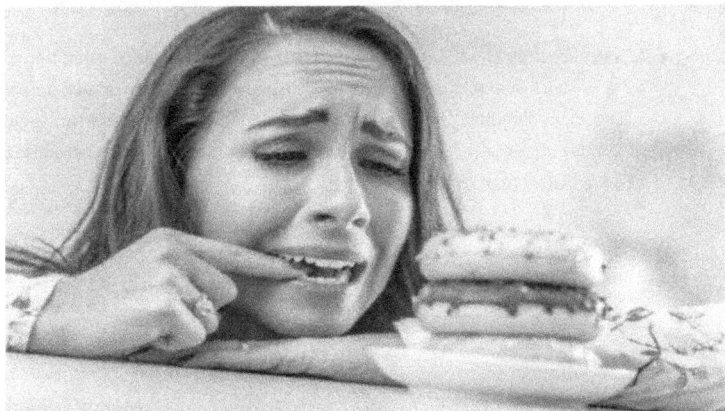

Here are some quick ADDED SUGAR facts for you:

- Most added sugar comes from prepared and processed foods.

- Soft drinks and breakfast cereals are the grocery staples that contain the most added sugars.
- The average soft drink can contain 150 calories, most of which come from high-fructose corn syrup. This is roughly the equivalent of 10 teaspoons of table sugar!

High fructose corn syrup, derived from *corn starch*, is way cheaper and sweeter than normal sugar. It's absorbed by the body faster (sugar rush!), and is linked to insulin resistance, obesity, Type 2 diabetes, and high blood pressure.

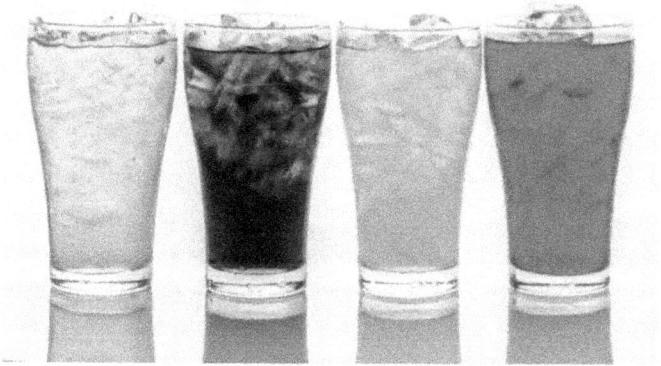

- The American Heart Association recommends added sugar consumption to be no more than 100 calories per day for women (6 teaspoons or 24 grams of sugar), and no more than 150 calories per day for men (9 teaspoons or 36 grams).[8] However, most Americans consume more than 19 teaspoons of added sugar (290 calories) per day!

HOT TIP: When buying something, quickly go over the nutritional label of the food item. If 'sugar' is listed as the first or second ingredient, then skip that product as you're basically just adding calories to your diet.

See also Appendix B for a list of the most common names for sugar.

Ok, so now you know that ADDED SUGAR is all around you and that's one of the reasons why you consume so much of it. Basically, you UNKNOWINGLY consume a lot of added sugar.

Another reason we consume so much added sugar is that research has shown that it's biologically addicting.[9]

Sugar causes **dopamine** to be released in the reward center of the brain. This response is similar to what addictive drugs do. If you consume a lot of sugar, you're reinforcing this 'reward' pattern, making it difficult to break such a habit.

Also ever wondered why you get such a 'rush' after eating candy, a cookie, or a piece of chocolate cake? This is because the added sugar in these food items quickly turns into glucose in your bloodstream, resulting in a 'sugar high'. However, the 'high' fizzles out fast and now you experience a sudden drop in energy. What do you do?

You look for more sweets to regain that 'sugar high'. So what you're really just doing is reinforcing a bad eating habit that's making you fat and unhealthy.

By the way, **sugar is NOT all about sweets**. Flour-based foods such as your favorite baked goods (donuts, pies, cake, white bread, pasta, etc.) are complex carbs that the body breaks down into simple sugars.

And sugar can 'hide' too. They may not taste sweet but items like ketchup, barbecue sauce, pasta sauce, flavored coffees, and reduced-fat salad dressings, can be high in sugar.

With all of the above, you're probably thinking...

Am I doomed to consume sugar? **No, you're not.**
Don't I have a choice? **Yes, you do.**
Can't I make a change? **Yes, you can!**

Following a zero sugar diet can retrain your taste buds so that you break that bad sugar habit! And in the process, I promise that you will live your best life yet.

Why Eliminate Added Sugar?

Oh boy, where do we start? Following are some of the known dangers of consuming too much added sugar.

Obesity

Studies show that those who follow **diets high in added sugar are more likely to develop obesity.**[10]

Studies show that high-sugar, high-carb diets lead to an unhealthy gut, which is one of the reasons for the development of obesity.

Also, unlike previous years, today's diet includes a lot of soda consumption. These drinks are high in sugar, which leads to a high-calorie intake. This doesn't only lead to weight gain, but to a decrease in the consumption of other important nutrients too!

Cancer

Research on lab rats found that a high-sugar diet may increase the development of breast cancer.

In another study involving more than 35,000 women, it was found that a high-sugar eating lifestyle nearly had twice the risk of developing colon cancer, compared to subjects who followed a diet with less added sugar.

The theory is that high (added) sugar intake leads to inflammation. And in the long-term, this sugar-caused inflammation damages the body's cells and its innate ability to fight off diseases.

Insulin Resistance

Studies show that when you consume more added sugar than you should, excess glucose is produced in the body. When this happens, **insulin resistance** occurs, which can lead to the development of **prediabetes**, and eventually **Type 2 diabetes**.

High insulin levels from consuming too much sugar are also believed to increase one's risk of developing cancer.

Oral Health

A **high sugar diet is also linked to bad oral health**[11] such as oral infections and ulcers, tooth decay, halitosis (bad breath), oral thrush, gum disease, and others.

Fatigue, stress and anxiety, joint pain, skin problems, acid reflux, and irritable bowel syndrome are also all linked to a high sugar diet.

As you can see, a high-sugar diet can wreak havoc on your health. If you adopt a zero sugar diet, you're not just addressing one health issue. You are managing and preventing A LOT of potential health problems.

What is the ZERO SUGAR diet?

In a nutshell, a zero sugar diet is an eating lifestyle wherein the focus is on consuming nutritious high-fiber foods, such as whole grains, fruits, vegetables, and nuts, as well as lean protein.

A sugar-free diet aims to 'flush out' sugar and its negative effects on your body completely. It will reset your brain back to the state when it was not craving sugar as much as you do now, breaking your body's dependence on it.

A zero sugar lifestyle also means you'll be FREE from the roller coaster sugar highs and lows that have a negative effect on your daily energy, mood, and waistline.

The Link Between Sugar and Carbs

As you go on a zero sugar eating lifestyle, you'll find that you automatically adopt a low carbohydrate diet as well. This is because carbs and sugar are linked to each other.

For starters, **sugars, starches, and fiber are carbohydrates.**

Complex Carbohydrates

Complex carbs contain naturally-occurring sugars that are harder to break down (in the body) and thus take longer to digest. And as mentioned above, a STEADY flow of sugar prevents sugar highs and crashes and is thus beneficial to weight loss and overall health.

Complex carbs also have prebiotic properties that support the growth of good bacteria in the gut. In addition, they are high in fiber and nutrients, which help to make us feel fuller for longer periods of time.

Simple Carbohydrates

Simple carbs are fast-digesting sugars. They can be present in complex carbohydrates, but they are mostly found in BIG quantities in processed foods. Processed foods often include refined sugars that are extracted and purified from plants, like sugar beets, sugar cane, and corn.

Simple carbs are NOT nutritious. And since they break down easily in the body, you don't feel full for longer. As a result, you reach out for these types of foods (again!) more easily. This, of course, leads to an excessive intake of calories.

Our body needs complex carbohydrates in order to function. The glucose they provide is the main fuel source for the brain and it's needed for proper muscle function. We don't need simple carbohydrates as they have little to no nutritional value. So, given the above, the best way to go low carbohydrate is to stick to complex carbs and get rid of simple carbs (or at the very least, limit your consumption of it).

The Effects of Going 'Low Carb' on Your Body

There are three macronutrients found in food.

1. **Carbohydrates** (4 kcal/gm)
2. **Fat** (9 kcal/gm)
3. **Protein** (4 kcal/gm)

As such, studies have defined 'low carbohydrate' as a percent of daily macronutrient intake or total daily carbohydrate load.[12] In particular:

- Very low carbohydrate (< 10% carbohydrates) or 20-50 gm/day
- **low carbohydrate (<26% carbohydrates) or less than < 130 gm/day**
- Moderate carbohydrate (26%-44%)
- High carbohydrate (45% or greater)

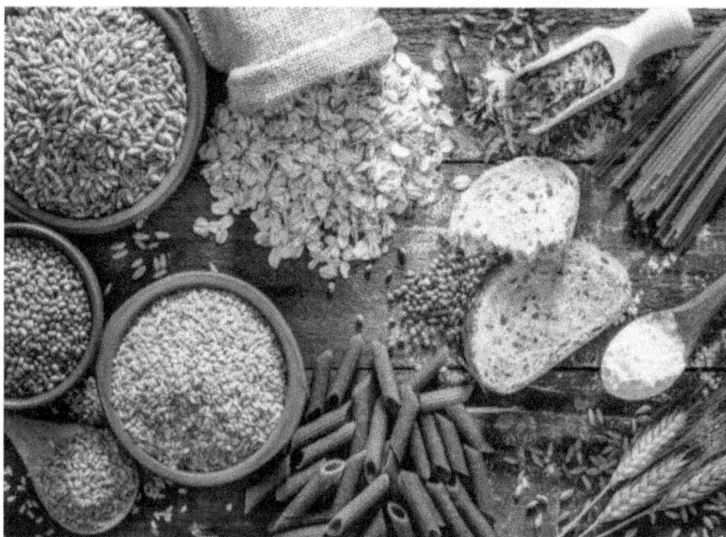

When you begin a low carbohydrate diet, your body will of course notice something different. It will be on a search for more sugar to burn for fuel.

Without getting the sugar it needs from food, your blood sugar levels will lower and your cortisol levels will rise. Cortisol is a hormone released by your adrenal glands to confirm you have enough energy to survive.

When your blood sugar levels are low, your brain sends a signal to your adrenal glands to release cortisol. The cortisol then starts a process called *gluconeogenesis*, which tells your body to convert protein and fat into sugar.

This is the stage low carbohydrate dieters want –> when the body starts to adapt by burning fat for fuel instead of protein. This is called ketosis.

Basically, ketosis is the body's method of ensuring you don't burn away muscle mass and glycogen during times of carbohydrate and/or protein restriction.

However, note that ketosis is NOT an overnight event. It can take a few days before your body enters into *ketosis*, which may leave you stressed, fatigued, and weak.

Now, you may be thinking... is it worth it?

To burn fat for fuel, should you go low on carbohydrates and put your body through all this 'stress'? Studies think so. One study showed that the increase in cortisol levels on a low carbohydrate diet was trivial when compared to the cortisol levels of people on moderate and high-carb diets.

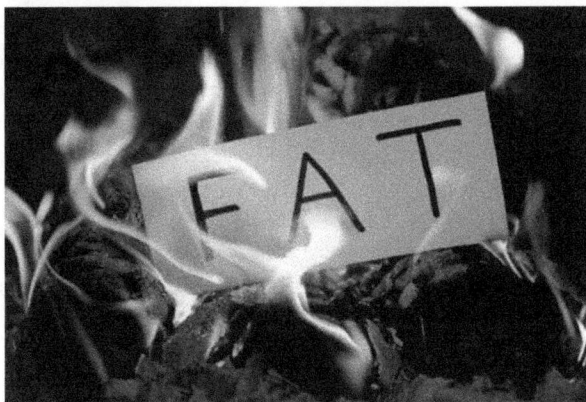

What other results can you expect from a low carbohydrate diet?

> **You'll feel less hungry.**
>
> What makes you feel full? What satiates hunger?
>
> Nutrients - fiber, protein, and healthy fats – make you feel full. Empty calories (from simple carbs and added sugars) do not satisfy hunger. So a low carbohydrate diet

> **You'll lose belly fat.**
>
> When you go low carbohydrate, your food choices tend to go high fiber. And that's a great thing! Most Americans on average consume only 15 grams of fiber daily, against the 19-38 grams per day recommended by the Institute of Medicine.[13]
>
> What's the connection? Fiber is needed by our healthy gut microbes. A diet rich in simple carbs and sugar promotes the growth of bad gut bacteria, which in turn promotes consistent bloating.

> **You'll build muscle.**
>
> Simple carbohydrates lack protein, the building blocks of muscle. By filling your body with protein and other nutrients, you're giving your muscles what it needs to develop without having to find additional calories. Also, an overweight body *covers* muscles with fat. But since you're burning fat in a low carbohydrate diet, your muscles will now have a chance to show. (Hello, toned body!)

> **You'll feel more energized.**
>
> Since you're consuming food that provides body fuel for longer periods of time, you'll have a steady - and non-fluctuating! - source of energy. Ever wondered why healthy people don't seem to ever go 'low bat'? This is the reason.

> **And of course, you'll lose weight!**
>
> If you follow a low carbohydrate diet well, your body will enter ketosis and burn stored fat. This is why low carbohydrate diets are seen as a means for rapid weight loss!

However, in the interest of completeness, note that going low on carbohydrates can also have some less-than-appealing side effects.

You see, ketosis is NOT an overnight event. It can take a few days before your body enters into ketosis, which can result in the following side effects.

- Headache/migraines
- Bad breath (halitosis)
- Weakness
- Fatigue
- Constipation or diarrhea
- Hair loss

Although some may experience the above negative side effects, many people on a low carbohydrate diet do not report them at all.

To be on the safe side, always consult a physician before embarking on any new dietary change. And be vigilant about your own body! Monitor how your body is reacting to changes and react accordingly.

Low Carbohydrate Diets and Hydration

When your carbohydrate intake is very low, the insulin levels in your body go low too. And when insulin is low, your liver starts to burn fat and make ketones (*ketosis*).

However, low insulin levels have other effects. Low insulin also results in water, sodium, and potassium loss through urine.[14] This means that a very low carbohydrate diet **increases your body's needs** for both fluids and electrolytes.

This is why some people tend to suffer from dehydration at the start of a very low carbohydrate diet. The lack of fluids results in cramps, **fatigue, and headaches... also** known as the *keto flu*.

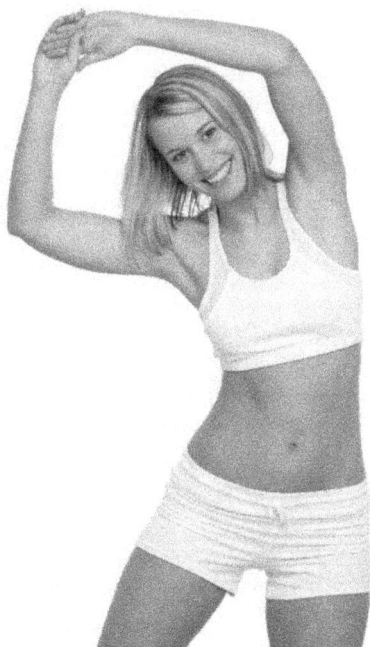

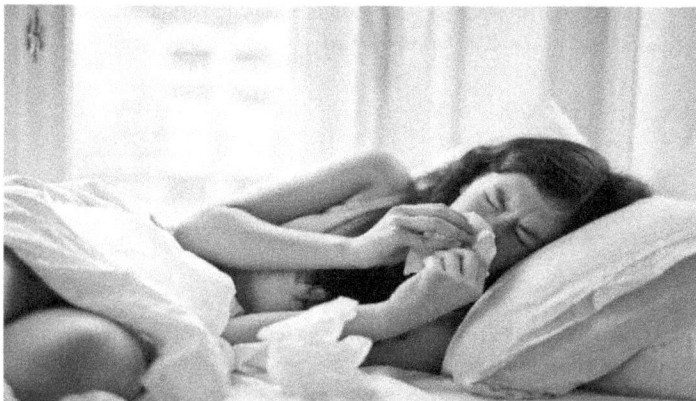

Now you may think that to battle keto flu, you should simply drink A LOT of water. Not quite.

Remember, you're losing water AND electrolytes. If you drink too much water, you run the risk of diluting blood sodium levels and thus boost the risk of *hyponatremia* (low sodium condition state).

So how do you stay properly hydrated on a low carbohydrate diet? Researchers believe in the following principles:

1. **Drink water when thirsty.**

   Here's a tip: if you get tired of drinking plain water, then drink fruit-flavored water. But don't just use any fruit as they may have a high glycemic load. (You will just be reversing the effects of your ketosis if you drink sugar-heavy drinks, even if they are natural sugars.) Use berries or citrus peels to flavor your water.

2. **Consume enough electrolytes.**

   Consume fluid-balancing electrolytes (sodium and potassium) through food and supplements. This means you should **eat a lot of potassium-rich leafy greens** such as Swiss chard, beet greens, lima beans, acorn squash, spinach, pakchoi (bok choy), white button mushrooms, tomatoes, Brussel sprouts, broccoli, green peas, and fennel.

   You should also **add a bit more salt to your food than you would normally consume**. Salt your eggs, your rice, meat, etc. The recommended daily limit on salt intake is 2.3 grams per day. However, since you're trying to up your electrolytes, you can consume around 5 grams of sodium per day (about 2.5 teaspoons of salt).

You may also **consider taking a high-quality supplement** that contains plenty of sodium. Ideally, a supplement with at least 500 mg of sodium per serving.

There's another reason to ensure you're properly hydrated during a low carbohydrate diet – *keto breath.*

The ketones produced in your body during ketosis are released through your breath as acetone. Some people report a fruity or sweet breath scent. Others, however, liken the breath to rotten apples or nail polish remover. And if you don't hydrate well, you'll suffer from a dry mouth, which means there's not enough saliva to remove bacteria and food particles in your mouth. So - stay hydrated!

And since keto breath is not at all sexy, here are more tips to avoid it.

➤ Improve oral hygiene.

In addition to brushing your teeth after each meal, consider the following oral hygiene practices too:

- **Floss away.** Flossing is a great way to get rid of food particles stuck between your teeth. You may already practice this before you sleep but consider doing it after every meal. You don't want those food particles to rot and cause even more unpleasant breath, do you?

- **Clean and scrape your tongue.** Consider buying a tongue scraper to rid your tongue of bacteria. One study found that tongue scraping twice a day for a week lowered the presence of *Mutans streptococci* and *Lactobacilli bacteria* in the mouth. These bacteria are credited to induce bad breath and tooth decay.[15]

- **Give 'oil pulling' a try.** Coconut oil is known for its antibacterial properties. To oil pull, swirl a small amount of coconut oil in your mouth and in between your teeth. This swishing 'pulls' unfriendly bacteria from your tongue, gums, cheek walls, etc., and gets eliminated when you spit.

➢ **Drink LEMON water.**

In addition to helping you replenish your electrolytes, lemons also contain antibacterial properties. So, you get hydrated and you rid your mouth of odor-causing bacteria.

➢ **Try natural breath fresheners.**

At the first sign of bad breath, you may want to turn to gum and fresh mints. Don't! These products are usually loaded with added sugars. Before you know it, you're out of ketosis faster than it took you to get to that state.

A better alternative is to turn to natural breath fresheners such as mint, sage, fennel seeds, parsley, cinnamon, clove, marjoram, and cardamom.

Don't want to chew the real thing? Look for all-natural extracts of these herbs and use them as a mouth spray.

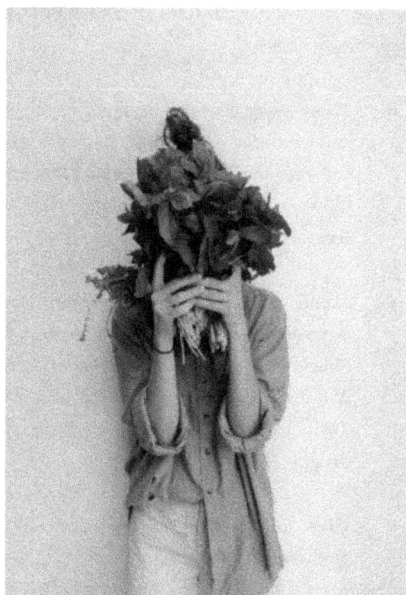

Chapter 3
How to Break Away from Sugar

Food Habits to Break Away from Sugar for Life

Eat breakfast.

Breakfast is important. However, it's not the act of having it that makes you lose weight; it's the choices you make.

Many people think that by skipping breakfast, they reduce calorie consumption and thus lose weight. However, what happens in REAL LIFE is that by skipping breakfast, you lower your blood sugar levels so much so that by the time lunch comes around, you're so hungry that you make the WRONG food choices.

So don't skip breakfast. Instead, have a healthy zero sugar breakfast!
(Click here for low carb, zero sugar breakfast recipes.)

Sweeten foods naturally yourself.

So many food items have added sugars that it's now hard to determine what food tastes like naturally. So go back to basics and sweeten foods yourself. This means mostly using fruit as your sweetener. Stevia, a plant-based natural sweetener may also be used. However, apart from these, stay away from other sugar substitutes. This is because some sugar substitutes mess with your metabolism and even induce hunger.

Also, slowly lessen the amount of natural sweetener you use. For instance, if you use three (3) teaspoons of stevia for your morning steel-cut oatmeal, lower this to two (2) teaspoons after a week.

Schedule your meals.

It's all about balance and trying to maintain your blood sugar levels at a stable, non-roller-coaster pace. To achieve this, you need to evenly space out and schedule your meals during the day. The general rule is to eat a healthy meal every three to four hours. Of course, you may not always be able to keep to a tight schedule. As such, always keep healthy snacks such as cut vegetables, dried fruit, and raw nuts and seeds with you.

Meticulously plan your meals.

Scheduling your meals will not give you an ounce of benefit if you're not eating the right foods so plan exactly what you should be eating in advance. Meal prepping is crucial here so that you're not tempted to choose something else. Also, ensure that there's a protein in each meal.

Tip: Don't know how to plan your meals, follow my detailed 7-Day Zero-Sugar Diet Eating Plan.

Learn appropriate serving sizes.
Quick! What does a single serving of grilled chicken look like? It's ok if you don't know, A LOT of people don't. However, the fact remains that we unconsciously overeat because we're not aware of proper serving sizes.

So here's a breakdown of common food items and their recommended single-serving sizes.

- **Grains**

1 slice (40g) of bread
½ medium (40g) roll or flatbread
½ cup (75-120g) cooked rice, pasta, noodles, barley, buckwheat, semolina, polenta, bulgur, or quinoa
½ cup (120g) cooked porridge
2/3 cup (30g) wheat cereal flakes
¼ cup (30g) muesli
3 (35g) crispbreads
1 (60g) crumpet
1 small (35g) English muffin or scone

- **Vegetables**

½ cup cooked vegetables
½ cup cooked dried or canned beans
1 cup green leafy or raw salad vegetables
½ cup sweet corn
½ medium sweet potato
1 medium tomato

- **Fruits**

1 medium apple, banana, orange, or pear
2 small apricots, kiwi fruits, or plums
1 cup diced or canned fruit (no added sugar)

- **Protein foods (meat, poultry, fish, dry beans, and nuts)**

65g cooked lean red meat (about 90-100g raw)

80g cooked lean poultry (about 100g raw)

100g cooked fish fillet (about 115g raw, or one small can of fish)

2 large (120g) eggs

1 cup (150g) cooked or canned legumes or beans (e.g., lentils, chickpeas, split peas, etc.)

170g tofu

30g nuts or seeds

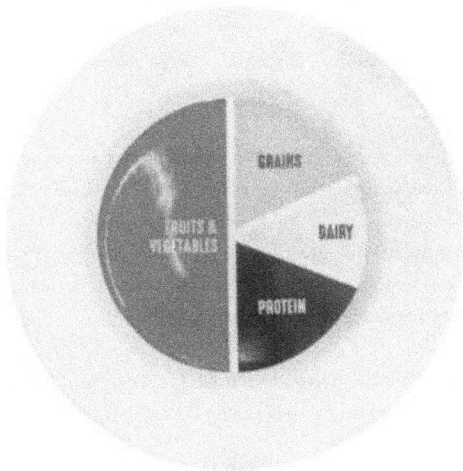

- **Dairy foods (milk, yogurt, and cheese)**

1 cup (250ml) fresh milk or buttermilk

2 slices (40g) hard cheese

½ cup (120g) ricotta cheese

¾ cup (200g) yogurt

1 cup (250ml) soy, rice, or other cereal drink

When you're at home, it's easy to keep track of the above. However, when eating out or at someone else's place, be guided visually by the following.

- One cup of raw leafy vegetables or a baked sweet potato should be around the size of a small fist.
- Three ounces of cooked poultry or lean meat should be around the size of a deck of cards.
- A teaspoon of soft margarine is about the size of a single die.
- An ounce and a half of fat-free or low-fat cheese are about the size of four stacked dice pieces.

Go for portion control.

Now that you know what a SINGLE serving of common food items is, how do you teach yourself not to go for more?

For starters, consider switching to a divided plate at home at the start of your weight loss journey.

This is just so you can get used to appropriate serving sizes. Soon enough, you'll find out that serving yourself the right amount will come naturally.

Follow the 20-minute rule. Think you're still hungry? Wait 20 minutes before going for a second serving. Studies show it takes about 20 minutes for the brain to get the message that you're full so wait it out a bit.

Learn the difference between REAL FOOD and FAKE FOOD.
Here are a couple of general rules on this.

- If nature didn't make it, it's not real food.
- If it's in a jar, packet, or box, it may be real food, but it's been processed so much that you might as well forget it because there's hardly any nutrients left. (Plus, added salt and sugar!)
- If there's something on the nutritional label that you can't pronounce, don't buy it.

Don't buy food, cook food.
We leave in a world where everything is ready-made. It may be convenient, but it also means we no longer have control over what we put in our mouths. However, do you really want food manufacturers to dictate what you eat? Take back your power by cooking your own food!

Also, buying cooked food or ready-to-eat meals come with a lot of salt, fat, and sugar. If you cook at home, you can avoid all of these. Here are some tips.

- **Steam vegetables.** When was the last time you were served 'virgin' side dishes in a restaurant? (The answer: never.) Steaming veggies at home means you get their full nutritional value, especially if you don't overcook them.
- **Don't deep-fry, bake, grill, or roast instead.** You already know deep-fried stuff is not good for you. Plus, if you bake, grill, or roast at home you have control over what marinade or sauce to use. (Go for low-fat liquids like broth, lemon juice, or even wine.)

- **Buy fish whole.** Not only is buying and steaming a whole fish more cost-effective, but it's also healthier because you skip all salt, sugar, and oil that come with pre-cooked or ready-to-eat fish meals.
- **Shop and cook with the changing seasons.** Buying foods in season is (1) healthier, (2) cheaper, (3) tastes better because they were not forced to ripen, and (4) it's pretty exciting to look forward to the different foods that each season brings!

How to Know If Your Body Is Getting Better

How do you know if the zero sugar diet is working for you? Although you can measure and keep track of your weight (after all, you just need a weight scale for that), I urge you to also take note of the many positive, healthy, life-altering changes that will happen while you're on this diet.

> You DON'T automatically reach out for unhealthy foods anymore.
Although it may be very hard to believe now, your desire for most of your current 'go-to' food items will disappear. While on the zero sugar diet, you'll learn techniques that will BREAK certain sugar addiction habits. As a result, you won't just instinctively reach for that cookie.

Weight loss alters your taste buds.[16] As you lose weight, your craving for certain food items will reduce or even disappear. Ever heard of formerly obese people gagging at the thought of eating foods they gorged on before? Well, that's all true and you'll experience it too.

> You DON'T think of food as an automatic reward for something anymore. From a very young age, we've been given food as a reward for something (e.g., good behavior, good grades, etc.). The minute you go for something else rather than food as a treat or prize for something great that happened to you - mark that event. That's one of the signs this diet is working for you.

> You sleep better and wake up differently.
Is tossing and turning in bed now a thing of the past? That's because weight loss is linked to improved sleep quality[17]. It's also related to a reduction in the occurrence of sleep apnea, a serious sleep disorder wherein you stop breathing at various intervals during sleep.

And guess what? Experiencing good quality sleep means you wake up refreshed, rejuvenated, and energized. This means no more dragging your feet out of bed, and struggling to find the energy to cope during the day.

➢ **Your hair and skin look different.**
It's not hype when someone says that you seem to be 'glowing' now that you've kicked sugar out of your life. As mentioned before, you are what you eat.

While you're on the zero sugar diet, the focus is on REAL FOOD that nourishes your entire body. And while not everyone will notice the positive changes inside your body, they won't be able to help but notice the differences outside it. The changes are primarily because of the vitamins and minerals you're now consuming. Also – water!

Water helps maintain clear skin and improve its elasticity, contributing to your younger look. In fact, drinking just two (2) cups of water can increase blood flow to your skin, giving it an even tone.

Water also reduces that 'puffy' look. Contrary to popular belief, puffiness is not a sign of excess water. It's a sign of dehydration!

When you're dehydrated, your skin KEEPS water. When you do drink enough water, your skin will 'let go' of this excess water and so your face will lose that swelling. puffy, or bloated look.

➢ **You'll be more mobile.**
Additional weight puts a lot of pressure on the knees and joints. In a 2012 study of adults with obesity and Type 2 diabetes, researchers found that as little as a 1% drop in weight made the subjects more mobile by over 7%![18]

So don't be surprised if things you thought were impossible for you to do before suddenly seem conceivable now.

➢ **You may find yourself not needing your meds.**
As you lose weight, your overall health improves. As a result, you may be able to take lower doses of your current medications or stop taking them altogether. That's a lot of savings for you! (As always, please check with your physician before you make any changes to your medications.)

➢ **You'll be more at peace with everything around you.**

Bad food means a bad mood. So many nasty chemicals are triggered in your brain due to bad and unhealthy food choices. Also, the constant sugar highs and lows do nothing for your mood. Hyper one moment, hangry (hungry + angry) the next is never attractive, no?

Overweight people also have a lot of insecurities[19] that are often masked as anger at everything and everyone. A deep sense of failure and unworthiness is also pretty common.

However, as you banish sugar and lose weight, you'll find yourself calmer, more relaxed, and more accepting of things and people around you.

➢ **Ok, your OLD clothes DON'T fit anymore!**

There is nothing to add to this, is there?

Chapter 4

Zero Sugar Diet Battle Plan

C HOOSING a healthy eating, healthy living lifestyle is one of the best decisions you'll ever make in your life. Many people do this but sadly, many people fail too because they are not armed with the right knowledge.

The following are practical, doable, REAL LIFE techniques to help you navigate certain crossroads you will definitely encounter in this journey.

7 Tips to Curb Your Sweet Tooth

Yes, resisting the urge to grab something sinfully sweet is hard but, repeat after me...IT CAN BE DONE!

1. **Brush your teeth.** Yep, when the craving hits, get up... and brush your teeth. Floss even! By altering the taste in your mouth, you shift your perspective. Also, have you ever tried to consume something immediately after brushing? The food or drink does not taste nice, no? This will serve to 'turn you off' those cravings sooner than you think.

2. **Water is your new best friend.** Are you hungry or thirsty? Believe it or not, it's sometimes hard to differentiate between a need for food and a need for hydration.

   This is because even a tiny amount of dehydration can activate the hypothalamus to turn on both the hunger and thirst centers of our brains. Drinking enough water is one of the easiest ways to keep sugar cravings at bay. Further, water consumption cuts down the chance of you reaching out for unhealthier beverages.

   10 Tips to Drink More Water!

   Believe it or not, many people find it hard to increase their water intake. You've probably already heard of the **8x8 rule** (eight 8-ounce glasses of water per day). That's just about two (2) liters of water. However, during a weight loss journey, it's recommended to increase this intake to three (3) liters per day, and a lot of people find this difficult.

- **Start your day with water.**

  When you wake up, start your day with a glass of lukewarm water (a slice of lemon in it wouldn't hurt either). Not only will this re-hydrate you after HOURS of zzzzz's but it's also a great way to stave off bingeing on the wrong type of breakfast.

- **Get an engaging water bottle.**

  Ok, this is personal. I've seen some grown-up women carry water bottles with designs of their favorite cartoon characters when they were little... in PINK! I say, good for you! Whatever it takes, right?

  However, if you don't want to go the nostalgic way, how about just the practical way? For instance, get a water bottle that's 'marked' with the different hours of the day so that you're reminded that you should drink a certain amount of water by, say, noon. (You can also just get an old water bottle and use a marker and write these hours down yourself.)

- **Get some rubber bands and put this around your drinking bottle.**

  Each time you finish, remove a rubber band from your drinking glass or bottle. Fill up and keep ongoing throughout the day till you remove all the rubber bands.

- **Flavor your water.**

  I get it; water can be so boring! Liven things up by slicing different fruits and putting them in your water. Lemon, mint, and ginger are personal favorites of mine. But feel free to experiment!

- **Spice it up.**

  Try eating spicy food that's BEYOND your comfort zone. It's guaranteed to make you reach for a glass of water. And you don't need to go out for this either. Start adding chili flakes, cayenne pepper, etc. to your dishes to up the ante. (This is great for your metabolism too!)

- **'Eat' water.**
  Snack on watermelons, cucumbers, celery, and so on.

- **1:1**
  Dining out or having an evening out? Drink a glass of water for every alcoholic and/or non-alcoholic beverage you consume.

- **Make water your 24/7 companion.**
  Make your water glass or bottle as close a companion as your mobile phone! Hey, if you carry it around, might as well make actual use of it, right?

- **High-tech it.**
  Download a water tracker app; preferable one that's constantly - irritatingly (i.e., something that constantly beeps till you take a sip of water).

- **End your day with water.**
  After brushing your teeth, grab a glass of water and drink. Bring the empty glass to your nightstand because, you know... you need it for tomorrow morning's first water sip :)

3. **Don't grab food, grab something inspirational.** One of the best ways to fight sugar cravings is to flood your mind with health and fitness-related inspiration instead.

For example, have you been taking notes of your weight loss journey? If you have, go and review your progress. See how far you've come. Be proud of that. Now is not the time to sabotage your progress, no?

Another example is to immediately grab a fitness magazine or visit a health and fitness website. Basically, instead of focusing on the craving, you're negating that by re-focusing on your health.

4. **Learn the art of 'healthy substituting'.**

    When the craving kicks – give in. However, give in with healthy substitutes!

    10 Healthy Substitutes for Common Snack Cravings

    - **Chocolate -> Dark chocolate.**

      Switch to organic dark chocolate (at least 70% pure). Dark chocolate is rich in nutrients and contains fiber, iron, magnesium, copper, potassium, phosphorus, zinc, and selenium. It's also rich in antioxidants.

    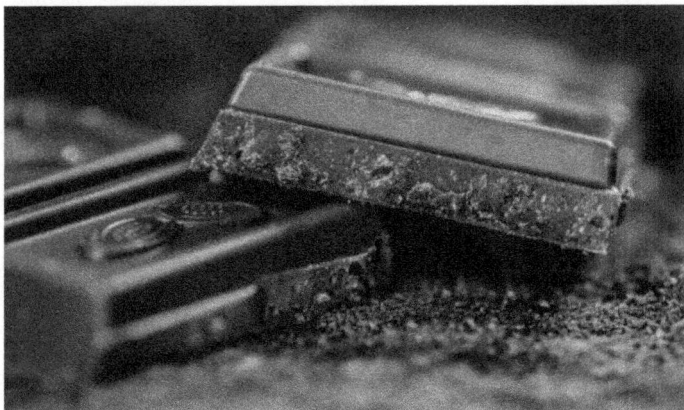

    - **Chips -> Baked sweet potato wedges; multi-grain flatbread with hummus**

      Sweet potatoes are rich in beta-carotene and have been proven to raise levels of vitamin A in our blood. They're also full of vitamins A[20], B6, C, and D. Vitamin B6 has been linked to helping decrease the concurrence of heart attacks and certain degenerative diseases. (Click here for a Baked Sweet Potato Wedges recipe.)

    - **Ice cream -> frozen, naturally-flavored flavored Greek yogurt.**

      Did you know that ice cream is basically churned frozen fat and sugar? Not good at all for healthy eating! Frozen yogurt, on the other hand, contains low levels of both and contains probiotics to help promote gut health. However, you will undo your good intentions if you flavor your yogurt with unhealthy food choices. The best is to mix it with fresh fruit and/or nuts. (Click here for a Greek yogurt ice cream recipe.)

- **Beer -> Red wine**
  Beer is high in calories. Depending on the type of beer, it can be anywhere from 200 to 400 per pint. The better alternative, if you must, is red wine, which has approximately 100-120 calories per glass. Red wine has also been linked to flavonoids, which may protect your skin from harmful UV rays.[21] Resveratrol in red wine may also reduce the effects of aging.

- **Hamburger -> Grilled chicken patty**
  The standard burger is about 350 calories. Grill a big, 150-gram piece of chicken breast, and you only consume 220 calories.

- **Pizza -> Whole wheat pita pockets.**
  Pizza, with its thick dough (starch!), layers of cheese (fat!), and unhealthy toppings (fat and salt!) may be delish but it's not healthy. Get the same satisfaction for less health damage with whole wheat pita bread stuffed with spicy grilled chicken, crunchy veggies, and a yogurt-based dressing.

- **Chips -> Popcorn**
  Potato chips, or any crisps for that matter, are loaded with salt and saturated fat. The problem too is that research has shown that consuming a very salty snack makes you crave and eat fatty foods in general, thus promoting weight gain.[22] So replace crisps with plain popcorn instead. They are full of antioxidants, fiber, and are low in calories.

  However, don't buy the flavored, buttered, already-popped variety as they contain a lot of salt and saturated fat too! Go for the unpopped corn kernels and pop them yourself.

- **Cake -> Whole wheat, organic banana bread**
  Cakes. Butter, flour, sugar... by now, you know this is not healthy eating, healthy living food. However, not all cakes are bad at all! Try this whole wheat, organic banana bread instead. It's rich in fiber and the whole wheat flour contains potassium, magnesium, and zinc.

- **Instant Noodles -> Homemade miso soup with buckwheat noodles**

  Apart from being salt city, a packet of instant noodles contains approximately 350 to 400 calories, plus about 14 grams of fat. Another problem is that instant noodles contain high levels of monosodium glutamate (MSG), a flavor enhancer that has been linked to having toxic effects on the body.[23]

  Try a homemade miso soup with buckwheat noodles instead. (Click here for a Miso Soup with Buckwheat Noodles recipe.) It's A LOT lower in calories. Plus, miso soup is known to have *A. oryzae*, a probiotic that's linked to lowering the risk of inflammatory bowel disease and other gut issues.

- **Cookie -> No-Bake Chocolate Cookie**

  Cookies. Butter, flour, sugar... They're just like cake - but harder. Reach for no-bake cookies instead. They are much lower in calories and since they're no-bake, they're easy to whip up too! (Click here for a No-Bake Chocolate Cookie recipe.)

5. **Break the pattern.**

   Most of the time, a craving is triggered by something. So instead of reacting automatically, by grabbing whatever it is you're craving, pause and ANALYZE the situation.

   - **What's the trigger?**

     Do you crave something every time you sit with your partner at the end of the day to unwind? If so, find an alternative non-food way to connect with your partner. This could simply be talking about each other's day, playing a board game or a hand of cards, or just talking about the kids and making plans.

     This is also a great opportunity to influence your partner to be healthier. For instance, instead of watching TV after dinner, encourage your partner to join you for a walk instead.

   - **PAUSE and find out what you really need.**

     A craving is sometimes not a need for food, but something else. Perhaps you're just thirsty, or you're unconsciously trying to put off doing something. Reflect and act on what you really need – not on the craving.

6. **Reach out – to your support group.**

Don't reach out for food, reach out for support. When you're going through something, you don't need a lecture, you need emotional support. So when a bad craving hits, hit up family, friends, colleagues, or an online support group who have gone through the same journey before.

They will understand better because they've already been through what you're going through. They will also be more equipped to help you overcome your cravings by giving 'been there, done that' advice, tips, or simply just by being there for you.

A Note About Lack of Support from Family and Close Friends

It's not uncommon to not get the help, support, and understanding you need from your immediate circle. Please have it in your heart not to blame them.

Firstly, **they don't want to lose you**. Food is a symbolic, social activity. We eat with family and friends to bond together. So a shift in how you see food may be extremely hard for them to understand. Most of the time though, it's really not about not wanting you to be healthy. It's about not understanding why you don't want to bond with them anymore.

Sadly though, this inability to understand you creates a situation where your healthy eating, healthy living attempts get sabotaged. For instance, your partner KNOWS you're trying to avoid late-night snacking and here he goes bringing out a sugar buffet of snacks.

Secondly, **they lack 'healthy eating' knowledge**. As you've read in this guide, sugar addiction is not just about sugar per se. It's about habits. It's about routine. It's about not knowing what sugar is doing to your body. It's about mindset. It's about knowing what to do to kick sugar to the curb.

#1 Greek Yogurt Ice CreamSo much knowledge is in your hands now; knowledge they don't have. As such, they don't understand, and thus can't support, the changes you want to make.

Thirdly, **they may be jealous of you**. Oftentimes, it's not just you struggling with weight and sugar addiction in your immediate circle. And any success you gain in your journey pricks at their conscience because now... you're leaving them behind.

So, the all-important question -> **what do you do?**
And here's the all-important answer -> **Live your life the way you want it!**

Remember that even though you understand why they may not or cannot support you, it doesn't mean that you should conform to what *they* want.
YOUR BODY. YOUR HEALTH. YOUR LIFE.
Don't follow them. Let them follow you!

7. **Wait for it to pass.** Sugar cravings come and go. The key is to wait it out. So the next time you feel the need for a sugar rush, hit pause. Take a deep breath and let it out slowly. Stand up and do something else. Ignore it. Yes, you can!

12 Sugar Addiction Battle Strategies

It's great to know how NOT to give in when sugar cravings hit, but isn't it better to avoid cravings altogether? You bet it is!

Here are 12 techniques to adapt to put a STOP to roller coaster cravings and binges.

#1 **Eat MINDFULLY.**
What does it mean to eat mindfully? I get this question a lot. Is it about meditating before you put any morsel of food in your body? No.

Mindful eating is about AWARENESS. Great! But how does that prevent sugar cravings and food addiction?

When you sit down to eat a meal, don't just chug it down. Take your time. Avoid distractions such as watching TV while you eat or staring blindly at your mobile device. You need to be in the moment to appreciate food and be satiated by it. And science supports this.

One study with binge eaters showed mindful eating lowered binge eating incidents from 4 to 1.5 times per week![24]

So basically, if you're MINDFUL or AWARE of food and how it nourishes your body, it's not likely that you will just go and grab something unhealthy.

5 Tips to Practice Mindful Eating

a) Eat and chew slowly.

b) Don't rush meals. Eating is not a contest.

c) Focus on the food or meal itself and ask yourself why it's a healthy choice.

d) Focus on the company. (Preferably eat meals with others.)

e) Before going for another serving, ask yourself first if you're REALLY still hungry.

#2 **Know your CRAVE O'CLOCK.**
We are creatures of habit. As you keep a food journal or simply take note of meal times and 'crave times', a pattern will emerge. If it's the dreaded 'post-lunch slump' of 'afternoon dip' – don't eat, take a nap! Studies show that taking afternoon naps boosts productivity[25] anyway so win-win!

#3 **Stock up on veggies.** Fibrous vegetables are low in calories and high in nutrients and fiber, so they fill you up longer, without introducing added calories into your system. Fruits and whole grains are of course healthy too but they are also rich in calories and usually have a higher glycemic load than their green, leafy counterparts. The moral lesson? Get most of your carbs from vegetables, and you PREVENT sugar cravings.

#4 **Stop looking at 'food porn'.** We are constantly bombarded with food pictures online. So, to prevent cravings from being triggered, avoid looking at food porn. If you must, then have a go-to list of websites and social media resources that focus on providing low carbohydrate, zero sugar food.

#5 **Hit the sack and get enough good-quality Zzzzzz.**
Sleep deprivation is linked to higher levels of body fat and appetite. Lack of good quality sleep also hinders cognitive function such as problem-solving, attentiveness, reasoning, and concentration. When you don't get enough sleep, you don't feel energized. You feel tired, grumpy, and hungry. And when you feel like this, your tendency is to crave foods high in sugar to artificially generate energy.

#6 **Learn techniques to overcome stress.** Life is full of stress - big and small. That's a given. Sadly, oftentimes, stress can lead to cravings. Somehow, somewhere, food has become a coping mechanism. So, let's learn some new ways to cope with the stress that has nothing to do with food.

15 Non-Food Related Ways to Deal with Every Stress

1. **BREATHE.** Deep breathing is one of the easiest and fastest ways to get rid of stress. When you breathe deeply, a message is sent to your brain to calm down and relax. The brain then sends this 'calm down' message to your body.
2. Read a **book.**
3. Play restful, **calming music** (e.g., rain, sounds of nature, etc.)
4. **Take a walk.**
5. Do **yoga.**
6. Take a 5- or 10-minute **meditation break.**
7. Take a **bath.**
8. Light a scented candle and **sit in silence.**
9. Go to YouTube and **watch funny videos.** Home videos, baby videos, animal videos, anything that will make you laugh.
10. Look at **family vacation pictures** or any picture that makes you feel happy. The point is to remind yourself of a happy point in your life to put your current stress into perspective.
11. Get your journal and **start writing** down (instead of acting on) your feelings. Journaling is a very powerful way to get rid of stress.

Many of the anti-stress tips here are about re-focusing the attention of your mind and body away from stress. Journaling, on the other hand, gives you a way to address stress directly.

For instance, you may want to shout at someone when stressed. Now, we both know that you might regret this action later so instead of ACTING on this urge, simply WRITE DOWN what you want to say to that person instead.

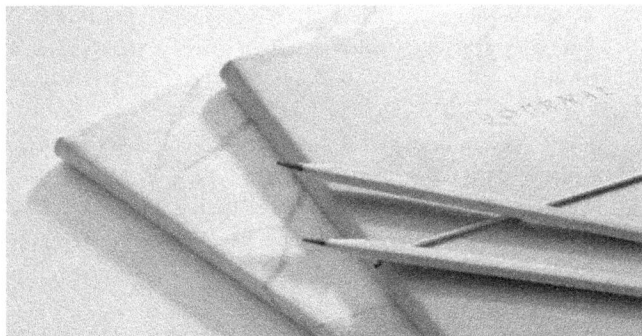

12. **Dance!** If the environment permits, play your favorite dance tune as loud as you can and stomp and shake the stress away.

13. **Call someone.**

14. **Work out.** Exercise releases endorphins, the happy hormone, and as such naturally reduces stress![26]

15. Don't ever forget this mantra – **THIS TOO WILL PASS.**

#7 **Eat more often.** It may sound counter-intuitive but spacing your meals every three or four hours prevents your blood sugar levels from dipping. As a result, you don't have those 'hunger pangs' and you won't reach out for a cookie for a 'quick fix'.

#8 **Spinach supplement, anyone?** Spinach supplements are now on the market and studies show that consuming 3.7–5 grams of spinach extract during meal times may lower appetite and cravings for several hours.[27]

#9 **Turn to vitamins.** If you're on a diet, chances are you may be lacking some important vitamin or mineral. This deficiency can also trigger the brain to activate its craving center so that you take in more food. The best way to handle this is to consult a physician before you start your weight loss journey and come up with a nutrition supplementation program to ensure you consume everything that your body needs.

#10 **You've got to move it, move it.** It is often said that you don't need to exercise to lose weight.[28] However, it's such a GREAT way to boost insulin sensitivity and speed up your metabolism. It may not be needed to lose weight, but it's definitely needed to be fit and to tone your body. And yes, it helps beat cravings!

#11 **Avoid boredom.** Oftentimes, sugar cravings are the result of boredom. Yes, there's such a thing as 'boredom eating'. There are two things you can do to avoid boredom.

Firstly, plan your days to a T. Grab your calendar, appointment notebook, or simply use your mobile phone and plan out every single hour of your day. This activity is called **block timing.** Keep in mind that you shouldn't fill your hours and days with just major events. The point is to plan and schedule everything so that there's absolutely no time to get bored.

For example, if you're usually free (and bored) after dinner till bedtime, then consider this.

Monday night: laundry!
Tuesday night: new hobby (e.g., cross-stitch, bullet journaling, etc.)
Wednesday night: call mom/brother/sister/friend/colleague
Thursday night: read a book or learn a new exercise routine
Friday night: me time (at least 1 hour soak in the tub; candles and all)
Saturday night: meal prep
Sunday night: plan coming week

Secondly, adopt a nighttime walk routine. Many people who can't find the time to exercise during the day find that walking at night enables them to get some movement in, and perhaps more importantly, enables them to have some ME time and reflect.

#12 **Don't go to the supermarket hungry!** When you're hungry while you do your grocery shopping, chances are you'll make unhealthy food choices. We go back again to that *instant gratification* or *instant fulfillment* we think we get by consuming high-calorie, sugar-laden food. Instead, have a 'shopping game plan' and stick to it.

Firstly, always have a grocery shopping list with you. Make it a habit to make your grocery list on a certain day (e.g., Sunday) and make it a habit to shop a certain day as well (e.g., Tuesday). This habit forces you to keep stock of what you have in-house and list only what you need for the week. When you shop, bring the list, and stick to it!

Secondly, know the layout of your grocery store. Once you know this, avoid all the 'unhealthy aisles', which are usually the middle aisles. When you enter the grocery store, spend most of your time on the produce section. This way, even if you're tempted to go to the middle aisles – you don't have time for it.

By the way, there's also research that hunger promotes the purchase of even non-food items.[29] So unless you need yet another potholder, don't shop hungry!

A Note on Dining Out and Handling Special Events
Going on a zero sugar diet doesn't mean you should skip going out altogether or miss important life events. As with grocery shopping, all you need is a game plan to address such situations.

• **Find out where you're eating out in advance**. Check out the menu beforehand, seek out the healthier options, and order these instead. Also, avoid consuming complementary food items set on the table such as breadsticks, salted nuts, white bread, and others as these are usually high-calorie, high-sugar food items. Opt to drink water with your meals too.

- **Go for appetizers.** Instead of ordering an appetizer and a main, consider ordering two appetizers instead. Also, ask for dressings on the side.

- **Ask for a healthy swap.** Luckily, many restaurants cater to healthy options nowadays, so instead of potato mash, ask if you can have a 'virgin' (nothing on it) baked sweet potato instead. Instead of white rice, ask for brown rice. If anything comes with a sauce, ask it to be served on the side.

- **Party time?** If you're going to a party where you KNOW there will be almost nothing but pizza, beer, and chips, then do the following: (1) Eat a light meal at home. (2) Arrive fashionably late! (3) DO NOT stand around the food table. (4) Socialize through conversion, not eating.

- <u>**Practice mindful eating.**</u>

- **Skip dessert.** Order black coffee or herb-infused tea and have a small piece of dark chocolate instead.

Clean Out Your Pantry, Freezer, and Refrigerator

Out of sight, out of mind. One of the best ways to succeed with your zero sugar diet is to simply remove temptation in your own house. After all, you can't deny yourself something, that's not there, right?

In one study, it was learned that people who had high-calorie foods within arm's reach are likely to weigh more than people who kept a bowl of fruit in their kitchens. [30] So to prevent any 'lapses', it's best if you clear out your pantry, freezer, and refrigerator of unhealthy food items before you embark on your zero sugar diet.

Look, chances are these places are up for some cleaning anyway; so take this as the perfect opportunity to declutter and organize these spaces.

As you go through these areas, you may find it hard to get rid of certain food items. You may even find it wasteful. However, remember this - your weight loss and health goals are far more important than holding onto comfort foods.

Think of it this way, you're not being wasteful. You're just getting rid of items that are making you sick.

Also, the goal is not just to empty your pantry, freezer, and refrigerator but to replenish them with items that you will need on hand during your zero sugar diet. As you will learn in Chapter 7, a zero sugar diet calls for making your own meals. Don't worry! All the recipes are easy and for beginners. You don't need to be a master chef to make them.

However, you'll soon realize that a new world of ingredients may be in order. And since you're just starting out, you may find it annoying to not have something in stock just when you're in the mood to meal prep. So, cleaning out your kitchen NOW is the perfect time to do it.

Tackling your refrigerator. Take everything out and give your refrigerator a good scrubbing (water + vinegar + washcloth will do).

What NOT to bring back: salad dressings, jams, soft drinks, and anything else that's high in calories and loaded with sugar.

Instead fill your ref with zero sugar essentials like cottage cheese, Greek yogurt, fruits, and vegetables. No time to dice and chop? Make life easier and buy pre-cut veggies and fruit.

Tackling your pantry. Same as with your refrigerator, take everything down and give your cupboards a good wipe. White bread, white rice, pasta, boxed macaroni and cheese, boxed breakfast cereals, bottled sauces... they all need to go. Don't be surprised if you find out there's hardly anything to put back.

In fact, I want you to take a **big step back and STARE at all the items you're going** to let go of. These are the things making you sick, fat, unhealthy, and unhappy. Be glad to let them go! And be excited about what you're going to replace them with.

Tip: For added 'excitement', think of recycling old jars or get some inexpensive transparent containers. Seeing your new food items on display can give such a healthy kick, and can be a real inspiration to get creative in the kitchen.

Tackling your freezer. Take out all freezer-burned items, frozen cakes and pastries, frozen dinners, frozen pizza, frozen snacks (I see you frozen cheese pockets!), and ice cream. What to bring back: frozen chicken, beef, fish, pork, and any other unprocessed meat option.

Although fresh is best, frozen fruits and vegetables are also great options to have in there. Frozen veggies can be quickly made into a great and healthy side dish, and frozen fruit can be quickly added to any healthy, energy-boosting smoothie.

HOW TO STOCK A LOW-SUGAR KITCHEN	
Clear Out	**Swap With**
Artificial sweeteners	Sugar/Stevia
Breakfast cereal	Oatmeal
Candy, dried fruit snack	Dark chocolate
Canned beans	Dried beans
Canned fruit	Fresh or frozen fruit
Canned vegetables	Fresh or frozen vegetables
Chip and crackers	Raw nuts (unsalted)
Crisps, chips	Popcorn
Egg substitutes	Eggs!
Fat-free yogurt	Greek yogurt
Flavored yogurt	Greek yogurt
Frozen dinners	Fresh meals
Fruit juice	Fruit-infused water
Margarine	Butter (preferably grass-fed)
Non-fat or skim milk	Whole milk
Processed cheese	Natural cheese (e.g., mozzarella, feta, cottage cheese)
Processed, canned meat	Lean cuts of meat
Protein or fiber bars	Fresh meals
Ready-made salad dressing	Homemade olive oil and lemon dressing
Soft drinks and sports drinks	Water, seltzer

oil	Vegetable oil/canola	Olive oil / Avocado oil / Extra-virgin olive oil
	White bread	Sprouted bread
	White pasta	Chickpea pasta
	White rice	Brown rice

Still not sure about what to clear out and what to keep? Here's a low-sugar kitchen list to guide you.

Tip: For the first few days of your zero sugar diet, it's best to have zero temptations in-house. Later on, you can buy tempting foods or snacks but then keep them on a higher shelf or anywhere that's NOT within easy reach.

<u>Think Beyond Your Kitchen</u>

Don't just focus on what's inside your kitchen. There are other ways you can support your new healthy eating, healthy living lifestyle.

Herb garden, anyone? Instead of buying dried herbs, why not have a steady supply of them by getting the real stuff? This saves money and you end up with a new hobby!

Go to your local garden nursery and select a few basic herbs to start with such as mint (natural breath freshener), basil (must-have in any pasta sauce), rosemary, thyme, and oregano. Go back home and re-pot or replant them in your garden. But if you're not up for a full garden just yet, then just keep the pots on your window sill or anywhere they can get ample sunshine. Take care of them and you'll be fully rewarded in turn!

Revisit your cookbooks. Dust off the cookbook shelf and get rid of (or store) anything related to baking and sugar. Instead, focus on cookbooks about healthy recipes. If you don't have any, no problem. No need to buy either. Just go online and start bookmarking healthy recipes, and make a deal with yourself to try at least one new zero-sugar recipe each week.

Improve your spice rack. On average, spices last up to three to four years. Anything longer should be thrown out. The exciting part now is replenishing your spice rack not just with new ones but with spices you've never tried before. After all, variety is the *spice* of life.

Weight Loss and Weight Maintenance

Losing weight is only half the battle. Maintaining your weight loss is the other half. The secret is to permanently adopt the healthy eating, healthy living activities you used during the diet.

A very low carbohydrate, zero sugar diet is used to jumpstart weight loss and break sugar's addictive claim on your mind and body. Once you've achieved this, you can slowly re-integrate carbs and sugar back into your diet.

However, it's imperative that you only add back COMPLEX CARBS and NATURAL SUGARS. Otherwise, you'll just be undoing all your hard work!

Check your calories. As mentioned before, with a zero sugar diet, you *automatically* decrease your calorie intake. However, for weight loss maintenance, it's a good idea to know how many calories you need to maintain your achieved weight.

There are many factors that affect your required calorie intake such as your age, gender, ethnicity, activity levels, and so on. You can use an online calculator to arrive at your daily caloric requirements. However, it's best to consult your physician.

Keep up the protein intake. Protein has been associated with improved metabolism, lower appetite, and supports certain weight-regulating hormones.[31] By continuing to focus on protein in your diet, you lower *ghrelin* (the hunger hormone) and improve *leptin* (the satiety hormone) in your body.

Also, protein takes more to break down in the body than carbs or fat. It's said that protein has a thermic effect of 20-30%, compared to carbs at 5-10%, and fat at 0-3%.[32] Protein is also believed to be great at suppressing cravings.

The bottom line is this: keep on focusing that you consume enough protein during meals for weight loss maintenance.

Weigh yourself regularly. This is a personal thing. Some people swear by it, while others claim to be stressed out by it. I say use it. Why? It's better to notice micro-changes in your weight so you don't overreact and overcompensate by making unhealthy and unsafe decisions such as skipping a meal.

Try to weigh yourself at the same time and day each week. However, choose 'weighing day' wisely. For instance, if Sunday is a family day celebrated with a BIG lunch or dinner, then skip Monday as your 'weighing day'. After such a meal, you're bound to be a bit heavier the following day. That's OK. You can't have the EXACT same weight every single day. Slight fluctuations occur. That's fine.

So choose your day and make it a habit to weigh yourself AFTER your morning bathroom rituals (but before your first meal of the day). If the scale says you're a bit heavier then take action by being more mindful of your food choice for a day or two.

The bottom line is this: treat the weighing scale as a useful tool, not an enemy.

Don't go back to the dark side. You've worked so hard. Wow, you! To *maintain* your weight, keep true to the healthy eating, healthy living principles you applied to *lose* weight.

MOVE ON. This is perhaps one of the best tips I can give you on weight loss maintenance. Many dieters fall prey to the thinking of 'going back' to old ways now that they've achieved their desired weight. On the contrary, what you should do is leave all that behind.

And it's not just about using the same techniques you learned to lose weight. It's about discovering NEW ways to motivate you on this road of healthy living.

Here are some examples:
- You learned that a support group can have a big, positive impact on your weight loss -> move on to supporting someone else.
- You learned how to set up a low-sugar kitchen -> move on to attending a low-sugar cooking class.
- You learned about smart food swaps -> move on to take complete stock of your life and see what other, better swaps you can do.

Chapter 5

A New Way of Eating = A New Way of Living

Identify Your 'DAY 1'

Y ou got the Healthy Eating for Healthy Living guide. That's a life-changing decision. Now it's time to further act on that decision by concretely deciding EXACTLY WHEN you should start your zero sugar life.

Some people just know that NOW is the perfect time. If you're one of them, go right ahead and complete this sentence.

I AM GOING TO START MY ZERO-SUGAR DIET ON: _____

Writing down an exact date is good because **you're committing to this change**, not to anyone, but **to YOURSELF**.

However, if you're not sure when the perfect time is, perhaps the following tips can help you.

➤ BEST 'DAY 1' TIP: After your birthday

According to research from the University of Pennsylvania[33], the day after your birthday is a great day to start to make BIG changes such as embarking on a health journey. This is called the 'fresh start' effect that many people feel after going through a personal milestone.

➤ BEST 'DAY 1' TIP: Monday

Mondays symbolize the start of the week, and as such may also symbolize the start of a new you. Also, Mondays are practical for many people because weekends are usually when family gatherings, birthday celebrations, and friend get-togethers happen.

➤ BEST 'DAY 1' TIP: Any day in October

This may sound counter-intuitive. After all, the holidays are just around the corner so are you setting yourself for failure? According to research[34], not at all.

The holidays do tend to make people gain weight. However, by starting a weight loss or health journey in October, you give yourself the opportunity to lose weight *before* the holidays. So even if you do gain some weight, you end up weighing the same (pre-October) once January rolls in.

On another note, many people who start a zero sugar diet in October find that they don't overindulge during the holidays. Why?

Firstly, they love what they've accomplished health- and weight-wise so they find it easy to 'stay true' to their new eating lifestyles.

Secondly, just as you've learned in this eBook, they now have the skills to eat mindfully and choose healthy food so quite frankly, unhealthy holiday food temptations are just not as strong as they used to!

Meal Planning and Meal Prepping

Meal planning is when you think about, plan, and list down the snacks and meals you want to consume in advance, preferable over the coming week (7 days).

Now, depending on your schedule and personal preference, you can simply plan out your meals and prep and cook them the day you plan to eat them or prepare and cook everything in advance (e.g., over the weekend), freeze them, and then thaw and reheat over the week.

Regardless of what option you choose, **meal planning is key to a zero sugar diet**. This way, you remove any possibility of grabbing snacks or meals that don't fit your zero sugar, low carbohydrate lifestyle.

How to Meal Plan

Deciding what to eat every single day can be stressful. And oftentimes, because life gets in the way, healthy meals are sacrificed in favor of 'something easy'.

Meal planning takes away a lot of the stress and pressure associated with answering this simple question - what do we eat today?

So, here's how to meal plan.

1. Pick a day of the week that's less hectic for you (e.g., Saturday afternoon or evening).

2. Take out a notebook and write down the coming days of the week; Monday thru Sunday. (You can also use a kitchen whiteboard so everyone can see the week's menu.)

3. Break down each day to Breakfast, Morning Snack, Lunch, Afternoon Snack, Dinner, and Dessert.

4. Keeping your zero sugar, low carbohydrate goals in mind, write down everything you should be eating for EACH meal.

5. Create a grocery list for the week based on your meal plan and stick to that list. No extras for now.

The advantage of meal planning is that you give yourself enough time to determine what you want to eat for the coming week. No stress.

Also, meal planning helps you come up with the RIGHT variety of healthy meals. During a busy week, you may not be realizing that you're eating the same meals (e.g., chicken and rice) over and over.

However, if you meal plan, you can mindfully choose what to eat over the mix and come up with a good, healthy, and nutritious variation of chicken, fish, meat, and vegetable meals.

Here's another tip: go online and look for zero sugar recipes you've never tried before. Go to Pinterest and search for yummy low carbohydrate ideas. Find zero sugar online forums and see what people are finding delicious. Let yourself be inspired!

How to Meal Prep

Let's face it. Even with the best intentions, a stressful day, feeling tired or unplanned events can lead to opting for the fast and easy solution – takeout or drive-thru.

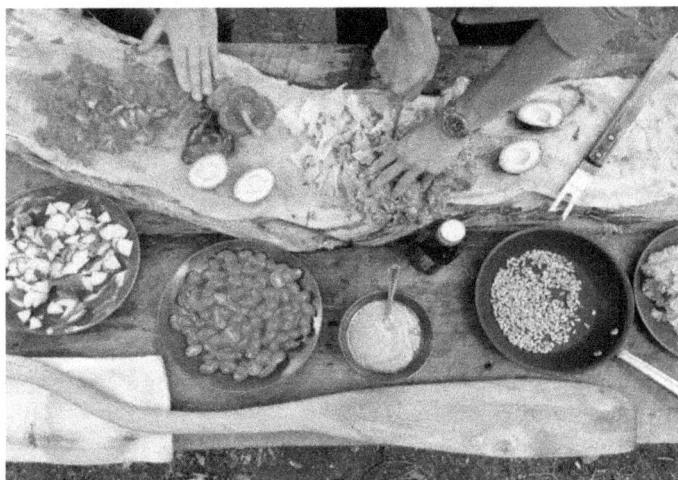

However, if you ALREADY have a tasty and healthy meal ready to be consumed… well, that's already 'fast food' right there!

Meal prepping is the next step to meal planning. It's acting on your healthy meal plans and intentions.

Meal prepping is when you prepare, cook, and portion out your emails in advance. Many people opt to make their meals on the weekend – Saturday or Sunday – and then put them in the freezer.

As the week progresses, you simply take out a frozen meal and let it thaw during the day or pop it directly in the microwave.

Is meal prepping tedious? It doesn't have to be!

Meal prepping can be a **fun family-bonding activity**. Get your partner and/or kids involved, and you just might be surprised at how much they like being a part of it.

Some people also like having **meal prepping get-togethers**, where a few friends cook together in large quantities and divide the resulting cooked food.

Whether you're doing it alone or with family and friends, here are some meal prepping methods for you:

- **Have ingredients ready-to-cook:** Cut, slice, and dice whatever you need for your planned meals. If necessary, steam, boil or bake them as well. On the day you need them, simply take them out of the fridge or freezer and cook away!

Example Recipe: Pasta Alla Norma

Ingredients:

2 eggplants, medium

1 onion, large

1 tbsp extra-virgin olive oil

2 cloves garlic, minced

1 can plum tomatoes

Salt and pepper to taste

Handful fresh basil (optional)

250 grams whole wheat or chickpea pasta

Directions:

1. **Weekend prep:** Pre-heat the oven to 200°C.
2. Chop the eggplants into bite-size pieces. Season it with salt and pepper and place them on a baking tray. (You can add other spices too such as oregano, chili flakes, etc.)
3. Bake the eggplants for 20-25 mins, tossing once.
4. In the meantime, chop the garlic and onion and put them into individual small containers.*
5. Take out the baked eggplants when done, cool, and refrigerate.
6. **Tuesday (or any weekday):** Cook the pasta as per package directions.
7. While waiting, sauté the pre-chopped garlic and onion until translucent.
8. Add the plum tomatoes. Season with salt and pepper.
9. Add the pre-baked eggplants and simmer until the pasta is cooked.
10. Add the pasta into the eggplant sauce. Toss and serve!

* **Tip:** If you use garlic and onion a lot in your meals, prepare a lot during the weekend and keep them (separately) in air-tight glass jars in the refrigerator. Saves a lot of time and stress during the week!

- **Make-ahead meals:** Prep and cook full meals over the weekend. Portion them out and freeze or refrigerate.

You can do this for the **Pasta Alla Norma** recipe above. Instead of cooking the whole meal on the day, you want to eat it. Cook the full meal on the weekend and simply reheat on the weekday.

- **Batch cooking:** This meal prepping method is great for meals that take longer to cook and use ingredients that freeze well.

For example, soups or meals that use beef take a long time to cook so instead of making just ONE family-sized portion, cook two or even three portions over the weekend. The meal can then be stored in the freezer and consumed over the coming weeks or even months.

- **Grab-and-go portions:** This method is great for snacks. Cut up A LOT of your favorite vegetables such as cucumbers, carrots, bell peppers, celery sticks, radishes, etc. Use a lunchbox or container with compartments and portion out a single serving of veggies, unsalted and unroasted nuts, and some fruit. Make a few of these grab-and-go treats to cover you over the weekdays. Handy AND healthy!

Figure out which meal prepping method suits you and your lifestyle and apply that one first. As you get more adept at meal prepping, trying the other methods should be easy.

As you may have noted above, meal prepping involves a lot of **FOOD STORING**.

Here are some tips on selecting the right storage containers.

- **Containers with compartments:** It's great if you can prep and put ingredients that belong to a specific meal together in one container. This means less searching for what you need when it's cooking time.

- **Airtight containers:** As you store ingredients and meals in the refrigerator, you don't want the various smells to co-mingle in there so it's best to keep them in airtight storage containers. Another advantage here is that they keep ingredients fresh and crisp longer.

- **Freezer-safe containers:** Prevent leakage, freezer burn, and loss of nutrients in your cooked meals by purchasing good-quality freezer-safe containers. Choose ones that stack well too to save freezer space.

☐ **BPA-free microwavable containers:** There's a lot of thawing and reheating when you meal prep so for your own health, invest in some quality BPA-free containers.

Lastly, to preserve the quality of planned meals and to prevent issues such as food poisoning, it's important to keep and reheat meals properly. Following are some important food safety standards from the USDA Food and Safety Inspection Service.[35]

✔ **Keep correct ref and freezer temperatures.**
Refrigerator temperatures should be kept at 5°C or below, while the freezer should be at -18°C) or below.

Tip: To be sure of refrigerator temps, get a fridge thermometer. They are inexpensive and help a lot in knowing the exact temperature of your refrigerator as you open and close it throughout the day.

Place the thermometer in different areas of your fridge every now and then to detect cold and warm spots. This way, you can position your food and drinks accordingly.

✔ **Cool foods before storing.**
After cooking certain ingredients or full meals, ensure you cool them down thoroughly before storing them. Cool them down fast by spreading them out on shallow containers and then pack and store them within two hours of cooking.

✔ **Label your meals,**
Apply a first in, first out approach to refrigerated cooked meals. This way, no meal is forgotten or stays longer in storage than it should. For this, it's best to label or mark your meals, i.e., write down the date you cooked the food.

✔ **Cook food to the right temperature.**
Invest in a food thermometer to ensure that food is cooked well. Most meats are cooked when their internal temperatures reach at least 75°C.

✔ **Thaw foods properly.**
When thawing prepared meals, it's best to take them out of the freezer a day ahead (or in the morning) and place them in the refrigerator. This enables the food to

defrost slowly and safely (less chance for bacteria to be introduced). Further, slow thawing helps preserve food structure.

If time does not permit this, dip frozen foods completely in a big container with cold tap water. Replace the water every 30 minutes.

✔ **Reheat meals at the right temperature.**
Cooked meals should be reheated to 75°C. Frozen meals should be thoroughly thawed, reheated, and then consumed within 24 hours after being defrosted. Do not refreeze!

Here's another tip: **discover new ways to cook food.**

It seems that today's diet is all about deep-drying. But did you know that the way you cook your food has a direct impact on how food affects your health? Deep frying, in particular, can cause potentially toxic compounds to be released, which can lead to heart disease, cancer, and other illnesses.

Now that you're exploring meal planning and meal prepping, it's the perfect time to discover the joys of other cooking methods.

- **Baking** is when you prepare food using dry heat, without direct exposure to flames, typically using an oven.

  Healthy example: Baked Sweet Potato
  - Preheat oven to 200°C.
  - Wash a sweet potato to get rid of any dirt.
  - Using a fork, poke holes around the sweet potato.
  - Wrap it in aluminum foil and place it in the preheated oven.
  - Bake for 45-55 minutes.

  Healthy example: Chicken en Papillote
  - Preheat oven to 200°C.
  - Take two boneless, skinless chicken thighs and place them on parchment paper.
  - Add any vegetables you have in your fridge such as cherry tomatoes, zucchini, mushrooms, etc.
  - Drizzle with extra-virgin olive oil, and season with salt and pepper.

- Bring the edges of the parchment paper to the center and fold them together tightly. Place the food packets on a sheet pan, and then place the sheet pan in the preheated oven.
- Bake for 20-25 minutes.

- **Broiling** is when you prepare food using direct, high heat. It's different from baking or roasting in that the food is turned during the process (usually midway) to cook either side at a time.

- **Poaching** is when you prepare food by simmering it with a small amount of liquid.

Healthy example: Poached Egg
- Crack an egg into a small bowl. Set aside.
- Bring a big pot of water to a boil, and then lower the heat to low.
- Add 1-2 tablespoons of vinegar to the water. Stir to create a vortex.
- Slowly add the egg to the middle of the vortex and cook it for 2-3 minutes.
- Using a slotted spoon, remove the egg and place it in some kitchen paper to remove any excess water.

- **Steaming** is when you prepare food by heating it in steam from boiling water. This is a great way of cooking vegetables as it preserves the flavor and a lot of its nutrients.

Healthy example: Steamed Green Beans
- Rinse the green beans and trim the edges.
- Put 1-2 inches of water in a medium to a large saucepan.
- Put a steamer basket on top of the saucepan, and place the green beans in the steamer basket.
- Bring the water to a boil. Reduce to medium-low, cover the saucepan, and steam the green beans for about 5 minutes.

*(Did you notice that we just made a whole meal with the **Chicken en Papillote**, **Baked Sweet Potato**, and the **Steamed Green Beans** recipes? Try it for dinner sometime!)*

- **Pressure cooking** is when you prepare food using a pressure cooker. This cooking method heats the air within a covered pot (the pressure cooker) to a

- very high temperature (above boiling point). This enables air pressure and steam to build up inside the cooking vessel, cooking food faster. As the pressure increases inside the pot, hot steam is compelled through the food to cook it thoroughly.

- **Simmering**, also known as the *moist heat method*, involves bringing water (or any liquid) to 85°C to 95°C (gentle bubbling) to cook food.

- **Stewing or slow cooking** is when you prepare food by subjecting it to a low temperature for a long period of time. Also known as the 'set it and forget it' cooking method, this technique is great for tendering tough meat cuts or when you simply don't have a lot of time to fuss in the kitchen. You can use either a slow cooker or your oven for this method.

- **Sous-vide** is when you prepare food by vacuum-sealing ingredients and immersing it in warm water. Just like slow cooking, it's a 'set it and forget it' cooking method. This is great for meal planning and prepping because you can pretty much put a whole meal in a vacuum pack, freeze it, and sous vide it during the week (without defrosting).

How to Shop for Healthy Food

Meal prepping starts with having healthy ingredients readily on hand in the kitchen. It's not surprising that changing your eating lifestyle also calls for a change in your grocery shopping habits. No worries though. I've got you covered with the following tips.

12 Tips to Help You Become Supermarket Savvy

1. Meal plan so that you can create an 'exact' grocery list.

   Tip: Don't just be a healthy shopper, be a savings savvy shopper too. Most grocery stores offer weekly discounts on certain food items. Focus on fresh produce, and keep this in mind when meal planning and creating your grocery list.

2. **Snack before you grocery shop.** When you're full, unhealthy food choices won't easily tempt you.

3. **Avoid free samples.** The supermarket is a breeding ground for many food marketers who want to introduce you to *What's New* in their assortment. Sadly,

most of these concern highly-manufactured food. So, skip the freebies and stay true to your low carbohydrate, zero sugar list.

4. **Send someone else to do the grocery shopping for you, preferably a man!** This may sound like an odd tip, but I swear it works. Men, in general, are not easily distracted by discounts, freebies, and free samples. They want to grab what's on the list and get out of there fast. So, if you know someone willing to do this for you – grab the opportunity.

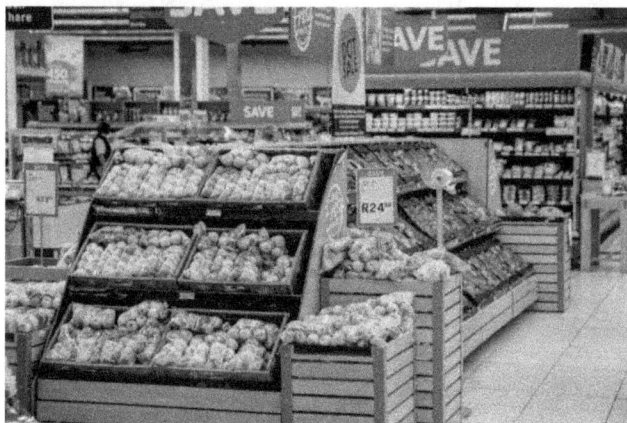

5. **Go for the rainbow.** Spend most of your time in the produce section and select fruits and vegetables of various colors. This is not just for aesthetics. The different colors represent the different vitamins and minerals you can get from each vegetable or fruit.

6. **Avoid anything that comes in a box or package.** These food items normally mean 'processed'. So, stay clear of these.

7. **There's no shame in pre-cut fruits and veggies.** If time is an issue when it comes to meal planning and prepping, do yourself a favor and go for pre-cut produce. They may cost a bit more but if it saves you time and stress, why not?

8. **Canned food can be good.** Fresh is best but canned food items such as tuna chunks in water and canned plum tomatoes are not bad at all. Just be sure you select canned food that's not processed with a ton of salt and sugar.

9.   **Avoid foods with hard-to-pronounce ingredients.** Real food is made up of easy-to-read and easy-to-understand ingredients. Once you see something on the label that's difficult to read or articulate, skip it.

10.   **Go beyond your local supermarket.** Instead of going to the supermarket, why not try and get the most of your week's supplies at the local farmer's market or food co-op? These places often offer the freshest seasonal produce, plenty of organic options, and many items sourced locally.

11.   **Buy in bulk.** If possible, stock up on healthy food choices so that you don't end up going to the supermarket often. For instance, whole grains like brown rice, steel-cut oats, dried beans, herbs and spices, and healthy snacks like popcorn can be bought in volume. This way, you don't need to constantly run to the supermarket and be tempted to grab something 'extra' on the way out.

However, don't panic buy. If you buy anything in bulk, do so for items that you KNOW you would normally consume during your zero sugar diet.

12.   **Switch to using sustainable bags, crates, and/or containers.** Apart from being planet-friendly, having a *specific* set of grocery bags and containers helps you curb any unwanted buying. If something unhealthy won't fit in your bag anymore, it doesn't belong there.

Chapter 6
Gut Health - The Anti-Candida Cleanse

Various types of fungi live inside and outside the body. This includes the genus of yeasts called *Candida*. In small amounts, *candida* is not a problem at all. However, when this yeast propagates uncontrollably, it can result in a yeast infection called *candidiasis*.

Thrush (Oropharyngeal Candidiasis)

Candida overgrowth in the mouth and throat is called *thrush*. It's common in newborn babies, seniors, and people with weakened immune systems.

Vaginal Candidiasis

Candida overgrowth in the vagina is called *vaginal candidiasis* and an estimated 1.4 million outpatient visits for vaginal candidiasis happen yearly in the US.[36] At best, vaginal thrush is an itchy, irritating inconvenience. However, if not properly addressed, it can become recurrent and lead to severe inflammation, or a serious skin infection.

Invasive Candidiasis

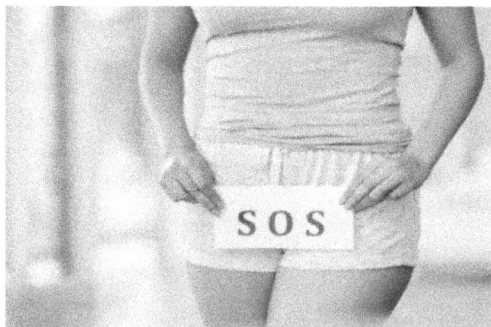

No matter where the yeast infection starts, if not treated properly, candida yeast can enter the bloodstream. It can traverse the heart, brain, blood, eyes, and bones. It is this scenario – *invasive candidiasis* – that can lead to a dangerous, life-threatening infection.

With the many problems that Candida overgrowth presents, it's not surprising for a Candida cleanse to be in order now and them. In addition to gut health benefits, a Candida cleanse is also beneficial for the following:

✔ Better food digestion.
✔ Lower inflammation in the body.
✔ Improved mood.
✔ Higher energy levels.

So it's important to always keep *candida* growth at normal levels. To do this, you should be mindful of what triggers candida overgrowth.

One of the reasons *candida* can grow uncontrollably is too much consumption of sugar, refined carbs, and processed foods.[37]

Anti-Candida Cleanse

Candida is a yeast infection. Sugar is the primary fuel source of yeast. For this reason, an anti-candida cleanse focuses on limiting the intake of food items that promote yeast growth.

On such a cleanse, flour-based food items, grains, and sweeteners should be avoided. Fruit and starchy vegetable intake should also be limited to two servings daily.

Here are some of the food items to CONSUME on an anti-candida cleanse.

✔ Avocado
✔ Bone broth
✔ Coconut oil
✔ Cruciferous vegetables (broccoli, cauliflower, cabbage, Brussels sprouts)
✔ Dark chocolate
✔ Eggs
✔ Ginger
✔ Grass-fed beef
✔ Herbs
✔ Leafy greens
✔ Lemon

- ✔ Non-starchy vegetables
- ✔ Nuts
- ✔ Olive oil and olives
- ✔ Pasture-raised poultry, including chicken
- ✔ Rooibos, green tea
- ✔ Seeds (e.g., chia seeds, flaxseed, etc._
- ✔ Some kinds of fruit, including tomatoes and berries like strawberries and raspberries
- ✔ Spices
- ✔ Water
- ✔ Wild fish

Here are some of the food items to AVOID on an anti-candida cleanse.

- ✘ Alcohol, particularly beer and other beverages fermented or made with yeast
- ✘ Dairy
- ✘ Fermented foods (yogurt, kefir, kimchi, kombucha, and sauerkraut)
- ✘ Flour-based foods (e.g., donuts, cakes, bread, bagels, pizza, etc.)
- ✘ Mushrooms
- ✘ High-sugar foods
- ✘ High-sugar beverages
- ✘ Vinegar, including apple cider vinegar

A Note on Gluten

Gluten has been linked to gut problems, inflammation issues, and Candida overgrowth. For this reason, it's important to steer clear of white bread, white pasta, and most cereals containing gluten. Instead focus on gluten-free grains such as buckwheat, quinoa, and millet.

Luckily, non-starchy veggies are naturally gluten-free so you can simply substitute certain vegetables for grains. For example, cauliflower and broccoli can be used to make *cauliflower rice* and *broccoli rice*. (Note: if you don't want to make a 100% switch, then do 50% brown rice + 50% cauliflower rice.) You can also use zucchini as a pasta substitute. (Click here for a Cauliflower Rice recipe.)

Further, you can substitute most flours for gluten-free alternatives, such as almond flour, chickpea flour, buckwheat flour, or even oatmeal flour!

Chapter 7

The 7-Day Zero Sugar Diet Eating Plan

Recipes make or break a diet. If it's too restrictive or if the food items are way too different from what you would normally consume, chances are, you lower your chances of sticking to your diet.

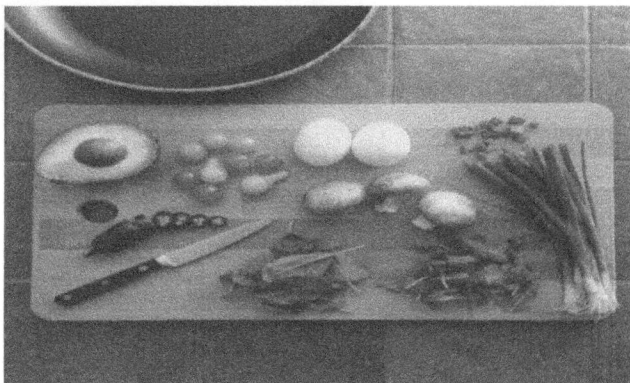

If your diet is composed mainly of 'bland food' that you need to eat over and over again, you won't stick to your diet either!

This is why I made sure to offer you a variety of recipes that fit the following criteria: delicious, easy to prepare, and made from easy-to-find ingredients.

By easy-to-find, I mean that they are readily available at most local supermarkets. However, I do concede that you may not be familiar with some of these ingredients. And for those particular items, this is what I ask of you – **please keep an open mind**.

Just because you're not familiar with something, it doesn't mean you shouldn't try it. Take this as the perfect opportunity to GROW your mind and food experience

The recipes are broken down into Breakfast, Lunch, Dinner, and Dessert and Snacks. And each category has seven (7) recipes. This way, you'll have a different – something to look forward to – delicious meal for each day of the week!

IMPORTANT: If you have any allergies, please search online for substitutes.

Breakfast Recipes

Mom's right. Breakfast is the most important meal of the day. This is the time you fuel your body and give it the nourishment and energy it needs to tackle the day ahead strongly and confidently.

#1   Power Cereal

Ingredients:

1/2 cup almonds, chopped

1/2 cup walnuts, chopped

1/2 cup unsweetened coconut flakes

1 tbsp sesame seeds

1 tbsp. chia seeds

1/2 tsp. ground clove

1/2 tsp. ground cinnamon

1 tsp. pure vanilla extract

1/2 tsp. kosher salt

1 large egg white

1/4 cup coconut oil, melted

Directions:

1.   Preheat your oven to 180°C degrees.
2.   In a bowl, mix the almonds, walnuts, coconut flakes, sesame seeds, and chia seeds.
3.   Add the cloves, cinnamon, vanilla, and salt.
4.   In a separate bowl, beat the egg white until foamy. Stir this into the granola mixture.
5.   Add the melted coconut oil to the mixture.
6.   Lightly grease a baking sheet, and pour the mixture over it, spreading it into an even layer.
7.   Bake for 20- 25 mins, or until golden brown. Stir halfway through.
8.   Cool before serving.

#2   Veggie Hash Browns

Ingredients:

1 large egg

1/4 tsp. garlic powder

1 cup shredded cabbage

1/4 small yellow onion, thinly sliced

1 tbsp. extra-virgin olive oil (or coconut oil or avocado oil)

Salt and pepper to taste

Directions:

1. Whisk together the egg garlic powder, salt, and pepper.
2. Add the shredded cabbage and onion into the egg mixture. Stir just to combine.
3. Heat the oil in a large skillet over medium heat.
4. Divide the hash mixture into two (2) patties on the pan.
5. Flatten them out a bit by pressing with a spatula.
6. Cook each side for about 3 minutes or until golden brown.
7. Serve with a slice of crispy bacon.

#3   Good Morning Sandwich

Ingredients:

2 egg whites

1 tbsp shredded cheese of your choice

1 tbsp chopped vegetable of your choice (e.g., carrot, green onion, spinach)

1 tbsp grilled turkey or chicken breast, chopped

Salt and pepper to taste

1 whole-wheat English muffin

Directions:

1. In a microwave-safe bowl, mix together all the ingredients apart from the English muffin. Microwave this mixture on high for 1 minute.
2. Take out and turn the egg mixture over and microwave for another 30 seconds to 1 minute.
3. In the meantime, slice and toast the English muffin.
4. Place the cooked egg mixture on the toasted English muffin.

#4   Beef, Spinach & Cheese Cups

Ingredients:

1 lb. ground beef

1 tbsp. thyme, chopped

2 cloves garlic, minced

1/2 tsp. paprika

1/2 tsp. ground cumin

1 1/2 cup spinach, chopped

½ cup white cheddar, shredded

12 quail eggs (if quail eggs are not available, use 12 small eggs)

1 tbsp. chives, chopped

Salt and pepper to taste

Directions:

1. Preheat oven to 180°C.
2. Lightly grease a muffin tin with cooking spray.
3. In a mixing bowl, mix together the ground beef with thyme, garlic, paprika, cumin, salt, and pepper.
4. Divide the mixture over the muffin tin. Press the mixture so that it goes up the sides to create a cup.
5. Divide the spinach and cheese evenly over the cups.
6. Crack an egg over the top of each cup.
7. Bake for about 25 minutes, or until the eggs are set and the beef mixture is cooked through.
8. Sprinkle the chives over the top just before serving.

#5 Cinnamon Overnight Oats

Ingredients:

50 grams steel-cut oats

1 tbsp chia seeds

1 tbsp dried dates, chopped

1 tbsp raisins

¼ tsp cinnamon

¼ tsp vanilla extract

160 ml almond or soy milk

80 g Greek yogurt, natural (unflavored)

Directions:

1. Get a clean jar (or any container) that will fit all the above ingredients.
2. Put all the ingredients in the order indicated above.
3. Cover and put in the fridge overnight.
4. Stir the next day and enjoy! (Note: if it's too dry for you, you can add a little more almond or soy milk.)

#6 Hearty Scrambled Eggs

Ingredients:

4 eggs, medium

1 tbsp grass-fed butter

2 cups spinach, chopped

1 clove garlic, minced

salt and pepper to taste

Directions:

1. Heat a pan on medium-high heat and melt the grass-fed butter.
2. In the meantime, crack and eggs in a bowl, add salt and pepper to taste, and then slightly scramble with a fork. Set aside.
3. Put the garlic in the pan and lightly sauté until softened.
4. Add the spinach and cook until just softened.
5. Add the eggs and scramble with a spatula or wooden spoon.
6. Remove the eggs from the heat. Optional: top with cheese and/or fresh herbs.

#7 Blueberry Pancakes

Ingredients:

1 cup whole-wheat flour

1 tsp baking powder

1/2 tsp baking soda

1/8 tsp salt

1 egg, lightly beaten

1 cup low-fat buttermilk

2 tbsp maple syrup alternatives: honey, agave sugar, coconut sugar)

Directions:

1. In a bowl, whisk together the whole-wheat flour, baking powder, baking soda, and salt.
2. In a separate bowl, mix together the egg, buttermilk, and maple syrup.
3. Push the dry ingredients to the side to create a well in the center.
4. Put the egg and buttermilk mixture in this space.
5. Heat a nonstick pan to medium-high heat. Smear some butter on the pan and then drop 1/4 cupful of the batter on the pan.
6. Cook until the edges begin to dry and bubbles appear at the top.
7. Flip and cook for a few minutes more.

Lunch Recipes

For your sugar-free, low carbohydrate mid-day meals, you want something that will boost your energy for the remainder of the day, without making you feel too full. Otherwise, your sugar levels will skyrocket and you'll start to feel an 'energy slump' by mid-afternoon.

So here are seven (7) lunch recipes that will give you just the right amount of energy and nourishment.

#1   Beef Taco Avocados

Ingredients:

4 avocados

1 lime

1 tbsp. EVOO (extra-virgin olive oil)

1 onion, small, chopped

1 lb. ground pork

1 packet low-sodium taco seasoning

Salt and pepper to taste

Toppings:

1 cup shredded cheese

1/2 cup shredded lettuce

Greek yogurt (alternative: cottage cheese)

Directions:

1. Cut the avocados in half and remove the pit.
2. Scoop out some of the avocado, creating a bigger 'cup' to hold the other ingredients.
3. Chop the avocado you removed. Squeeze a bit of lime juice over them so that they don't discolor. Set aside.
4. Heat a pan or skillet over medium heat. Add (or spray) some EVOO.
5. Add the onion to the pan and cook until softened.
6. Add the ground beef and low-sodium taco seasoning. Season with salt and pepper, and cook the meat for about 6-7 minutes.
7. Remove from heat and drain the fat.
8. Fill each avocado half with the taco beef mixture.
9. Top each mixture with the remaining cut avocado, cheese, lettuce, and Greek yogurt.

#2   Buffalo Shrimp Lettuce Wraps

Ingredients:

1/4 tbsp. butter

2 garlic cloves, minced

1/4 cup hot sauce

1 tbsp. EVOO (extra-virgin olive oil)

1 lb. shrimp, peeled and deveined

Salt and pepper to taste

1 head iceberg lettuce, leaves separated and washed (for serving)

1/4 red onion, finely chopped

1 rib celery, sliced thin

1/2 cup blue cheese, crumbled

Directions:

Buffalo sauce:

1. Melt the butter in a saucepan over medium heat.
2. Add the garlic and cook until fragrant.
3. Add the hot sauce to the garlic butter and stir
4. Turn the heat to low.

Shrimp sauté:

1. In a separate skillet or pan, heat some oil over medium heat.
2. Add the shrimp to the pan and season with salt and pepper.
3. Cook the shrimps until they turn pink and opaque.
4. Turn off the heat and add the Buffalo sauce to the shrimp mixture in the skillet. Toss to coat the shrimp.

Assembly:

1. Get an iceberg lettuce leaf. Add a scoop of shrimp, and then top with red onion, celery, and blue cheese.

#3   Yummy Cauliflower Salad

Ingredients:

1 medium-sized cauliflower, cut into florets

6 slices bacon

1/2 cup Greek yogurt

1/4 cup full-fat mayonnaise

1 tbsp. lemon juice

1/2 tsp. garlic powder

1 1/2 cup cheddar, shredded

1/4 cup chives, chopped

Directions:

1. Boil some water and then add the cauliflower florets.
2. Steam the cauliflower for about 4 minutes, or just until fork-tender.
3. Drain the cauliflower and set it aside to cool.
4. Heat a non-stick pan over medium heat. Add the bacon and cook until crispy.
5. Transfer the bacon to a paper towel-lined plate to drain excess fat. Once cool to handle, roughly chop the bacon.
6. Mix together the Greek yogurt, mayonnaise, lemon juice, and garlic powder in a bowl.
7. Add the steamed cauliflower and toss gently. Season with salt and pepper.
8. Add in the bacon, cheddar, and chives.

#4   Tuna and Zucchini Cakes

Ingredients:

1 can tuna

1 medium zucchini

1 medium white onion, shredded (or sliced very thinly)

1 small carrot, finely chopped

Salt and pepper to taste

¼ tsp smoked paprika

2 large eggs, lightly beaten

1 tbsp whole wheat bread crumbs

Butter for frying

Directions:

1. Open the tuna can and drain to get rid of excess liquid. Set aside.
2. Shred the zucchini. Squeeze out as much excess liquid as you can.
3. In a bowl, add the tuna, zucchini, white onion, carrot, salt and pepper, paprika, and lightly beaten eggs. Mix gently to combine.
4. Shape the mixture into 1/2-inch thick patties
5. Coat each patty in bread crumbs.
6. Heat a non-stick pan over medium-high heat. Add some butter.
7. Once the butter is melted, add the patties in batches so that they don't overcrowd the pan.
8. Cook about 3-5 minutes on each side or until golden brown and the zucchini is cooked through.

#5   Pizza!

Ingredients:
1 whole-wheat pita

1/2 cup low-sodium tomato sauce

1/4 cup shredded mozzarella

1/2 cup grilled chicken or turkey breast

1/4 cup chopped sun-dried tomatoes

Garlic and oregano to taste

Salt and pepper to taste

Directions:
1. Lightly toast the whole wheat pita bread.
2. Take the pita bread out and top with 1 tbsp of tomato sauce.
3. Add the rest of the toppings.
4. Sprinkle with garlic and oregano,
5. Place the pita back in the oven, put on 'broil' or 'grill' if possible, until the cheese bubbles.

#6   Spicy Tomato Soup

Ingredients:
1 tbsp butter

1 small white onion, chopped

2 cloves garlic, minced

1 tsp smoked paprika

4 medium tomatoes, chopped

1 cup chicken broth

1/2 cup cream cheese

salt and pepper to taste

fresh basil, optional for topping

Directions:
1. Place a saucepan over medium-high heat. Melt the butter.
2. Add the onion and garlic, and cook until fragrant and the onion is translucent.
3. Add the tomatoes to the saucepan. Cook just until the tomatoes are soft.
4. Add the chicken broth or stock to the pot and season with salt and pepper to taste.
5. Bring everything to a simmer, and then lower the heat to medium-low. Simmer the soup for about 10 minutes.
6. Turn off the heat.

7. Puree the soup using a stick or immersion blender until your desired consistency.
8. Optional: if you like your soup fine and without any 'bits', you can pass the soup through a fine sieve.
9. Add the cream cheese to the soup and stir to dissolve.
10. Ladle the soup into bowls, and garnish with lightly chopped fresh basil.

#7   It's A Wrap!

Ingredients:

2 large eggs

1/2 teaspoon hot sauce

Salt and pepper to taste

1 tbsp scallions, chopped

1 tbsp parsley, chopped

2 tbsp black bean dip

1 9-inch whole-wheat tortilla wrap

1 tsp extra-virgin olive oil

2 tbsp cheddar cheese, shredded

1 tbsp green or red salsa (optional)

Directions:

1. Set your oven to 'broil'.
2. Mix the eggs, hot sauce, salt and pepper, scallions, and parsley.
3. If the black bean dip is cold, warm it up first in the microwave for a few seconds.
4. Place the tortilla wrap between paper towels and warm in the microwave for a few seconds.
5. Spread the warmed black bean dip over the wrap.
6. Heat up a non-stick pan and brush some oil over it.
7. Add the egg mixture and cook through.
8. Place the skillet under the broiler and broil just until the top of the egg mixture is set.
9. Slide the omelet on top of the wrap. Sprinkle with cheddar cheese.
10. Roll the wrap and serve with salsa on the side (if using).

Dinner Recipes

Like many people, you probably look forward to a good dinner as a great way to end the day. Unfortunately, this is also why many tend to overeat at night. It's seen as a 'reward' after a tiring day.

Hopefully, after you try the breakfast and lunch recipes above, you'll soon discover that you don't head to dinner feeling starved and lacking energy. In fact, you might even feel the opposite and find yourself not wanting to eat as much as you used to during dinner time. Don't be surprised by this!

The recipes in this Healthy Eating for Healthy Living eBook are all designed to give you the RIGHT amount of energy throughout the day. No erratic energy highs and lows that lead to cravings, hunger pangs, and bingeing. So, let's get dinner cooking!

#1   Delish Mac & Cheese

Ingredients:

2 heads cauliflower, medium-sized, cut into florets

2 tbsp butter

1 cup heavy cream

150 grams cream cheese

4 cups cheddar, shredded

2 cups mozzarella, shredded

Salt and pepper to taste

Topping:

100 grams pork rinds, crushed

1/4 cup freshly grated Parmesan

1 tbsp extra-virgin olive oil

2 tbsp parsley, chopped for garnish

Directions:

1.   Preheat the oven to 190°C.
2.   Spray a 9x13-inch baking dish with cooking spray (or lightly butter it). Set aside.
3.   In a big bowl, add the cauliflower florets and two tablespoons of oil. Season with salt and pepper and toss.
4.   Spread the cauliflower onto two baking sheets. Roast them for about 40 minutes.
5.   While waiting for the cauliflower, warm the cream cheese in a big saucepan over medium heat.
6.   Once the cream cheese simmers, lower the heat to low.
7.   Add the cheddar and mozzarella cheeses. Stir until just melted, and then turn off the heat.
8.   Add the hot sauce and season the cheese mixture with salt and pepper.
9.   Add the roasted cauliflower, and toss gently.
10. Move the cauliflower and cheese mixture onto the prepared baking dish.

11. Combine the pork rinds, parmesan, and oil in a medium bowl, and sprinkle this on top of the cauliflower and cheese mixture.
12. Bake for about 15 minutes, or until the top becomes crusty and golden.
13. Take out and garnish with parsley.

#2   Southern 'Fried' Chicken

Ingredients:

4-5 bone-in, skin-on chicken thighs (about 1 kilo)

salt and pepper to taste

2 large eggs

1/2 cup heavy cream

3/4 cup almond flour

1 1/2 cup pork rinds, crushed

1/2 cup Parmesan, grated

1 tsp. garlic powder

1/2 tsp smoked paprika

1/2 cup mayonnaise

1 1/2 tsp hot sauce

Directions:

1. Preheat oven to 200°C.
2. Place parchment paper n a big baking sheet.
3. Pat the chicken thighs dry using paper towels and then season with salt and pepper.
4. Whisk the eggs and heavy cream together in a bowl.
5. In another bowl, mix together the almond flour, pork rinds, parmesan, garlic powder, and smoked paprika. Season with salt and pepper.
6. Dip the chicken pieces one at a time into the egg mixture, and then into the almond flour mixture.
7. Press the chicken pieces a bit into the almond flour to ensure they're properly coated. Place each coated chicken piece on the baking sheet.
8. Bake for about 45 minutes, or until the chicken register an internal temperature of 74°C.
9. Meanwhile, mix together the mayonnaise and hot sauce in a small bowl. Serve on the side with the 'fried' chicken.

#3   Miso Noodles With Chicken

Ingredients:

3/4 lb boneless, skinless chicken thighs

1 tbsp extra-virgin olive oil

1   bag   of   Japanese   buckwheat   soba   noodles

1/4 cup Shiro miso paste

1 tbsp low-sodium soy sauce

2 cups chicken or vegetable broth

5 stalks spring onions, sliced

1 tbsp sesame seeds, roasted

Directions:

1. Thinly slice the chicken thighs. Season with salt and pepper.
2. Put a non-stick pan on medium-low heat. Add the oil.
3. Sauté the chicken pieces until cooked. Set aside.
4. Cook the Japanese buckwheat soba noodles according to package directions. Set aside.
5. In a saucepan, put the Shiro miso paste, soy sauce, chicken or vegetable broth, and spring onions to a gentle simmer.
6. In a serving bowl, put the cooked chicken and drained soba noodles. Toss everything to combine.
7. Ladle the miso soup over the bowls.
8. Top with sliced spring onions and the roasted sesame seeds.

#4   Veggie Chili

Ingredients:

1 tbsp extra-virgin olive oil

1 small onion, chopped

3 cloves garlic, finely chopped

1 small green bell pepper, chopped

1 small red bell pepper, chopped

3/4 cup celery, chopped

3/4 cup dry red wine (or water)

2 cans diced tomatoes, undrained

1/4 cup tomato paste

2 cups vegetable stock

1 tbsp fresh cilantro, chopped

1 tbsp chili powder

1/2 tsp cumin

2 cans kidney beans, rinsed and drained

Directions:

1. Heat a large pan over medium-high heat. Add the butter.
2. Add the onion and garlic and cook until translucent.
3. Stir in the green and red bell peppers, and celery.
4. Add the wine and bring everything to a simmer.
5. Add the tomatoes (with juice), tomato paste, vegetable stock, cilantro, chili powder, and cumin. Stir.
6. Add in the kidney beans. Bring to a boil.
7. Reduce the heat to low, cover, and cook, stirring occasionally, for about 45 minutes.

#5   Steak w/Salsa Sauce

Ingredients:

2 4-ounce, 1/2-inch-thick steaks (e.g., rib-eye)

1 tsp chili powder

Salt and pepper to taste

1 tsp extra-virgin olive oil

2 large tomatoes, diced

2 tsp lime juice

1 tbsp fresh cilantro, chopped

Directions:

1. Trim the fat off the steaks.
2. Rub both sides of the steak with chili powder, and salt and pepper.
3. Heat the oil in a medium skillet (or grill pan) over medium-high heat.
4. Add the steaks and grill, turning once until it the met reaches your preferred level of doneness.
5. Put the steaks on a plate and cover them with foil. Let it rest while you make prepare the salsa.
6. Using the same skillet, add the tomatoes, lime juice, salt, and pepper.
7. Cook until the tomatoes soften.
8. In a bowl, put together the tomato salsa, cilantro, and, if you like, the juices from the steak.
9. Serve the steaks with the salsa on top.

#6   Mushroom and Scallion Chicken

Ingredients:

1 cup brown rice, cooked

100 grams shiitake mushrooms

250 grams boneless, skinless chicken thighs

salt and pepper to taste

1 tbsp sesame oil

1 garlic clove, finely chopped

2 cups water

2 tbsp cup low-sodium soy sauce

1 2-inch piece ginger, thinly sliced

3 stalks spring onions, sliced

Directions:

1. Remove the stems from the shiitake mushrooms. Slice the mushroom caps thinly and set them aside.
2. Slice the chicken thighs thinly. Season with salt and pepper. Set aside.
3. In a big pot, heat the sesame oil over medium-low heat.
4. Add the garlic and cook until fragrant.
5. Add the shiitake mushrooms and cook until softened.
6. Pour the water into the pot, and then add the soy sauce and ginger. Bring to a simmer. (Alternatively, you can use low-sodium chicken or vegetable broth. However, if you do this, reduce or completely omit the amount of soy sauce.)
7. Add the chicken into the broth. Reduce the heat to low, cover, and then let the chicken poach until it's just cooked through.
8. Divide the cooked brown rice over two bowls.
9. Divide the chicken over the bowls. Pour the broth over the chicken, and garnish with spring onions.

#7   Sunday Meatballs

Ingredients:

1 lb ground beef

1 clove garlic, minced

1/2 cup mozzarella, shredded

1/4 cup Parmesan, grated

2 tbsp. parsley, chopped

1 large egg, beaten

Salt and pepper to taste

2 tbsp extra-virgin olive oil

1 medium onion, chopped

2 cloves garlic, minced

1 can crushed tomatoes

1 tsp dried oregano

Directions:

1. In a big bowl, mix together the beef, garlic, mozzarella, parmesan, parsley, egg, salt, and pepper.
2. Form about 15-16 meatballs from the mixture. Place the meatballs in the refrigerator for about 30 mins. (This will help keep its shape while cooking.)
3. Heat the oil in a skillet over medium-high heat.
4. Add the meatballs to the skillet, turning occasionally, and cook for around 10 minutes
5. Remove the cooked meatballs and place them on a plate.
6. In the same skillet, put the garlic and onion and cook until the latter is soft and translucent.
7. Put in the tomatoes and oregano.
8. Put back the meatballs. Season with salt and pepper, cover, and simmer for 12-15 minutes or just until the sauce has thickened.

Dessert & Snack Ideas

Just because you're on a sugar-free, low carbohydrate diet doesn't mean you should deprive yourself of yummy snacks and desserts! Try the following treats and be surprised at how satisfying they can be.

#2

Ingredients:

2 cups of Greek yogurt, unsweetened and unflavored
1 cup strawberries, frozen
1 cup mixed berries, frozen
1 tsp vanilla extract
1 tbsp honey or maple syrup

Directions:

1. Put all the ingredients in a food processor, and process everything until creamy.
2. Serve the ice cream immediately or put it in an airtight container and freeze until ready to serve.

#3   Mocha Chia Pudding

Ingredients:

1 tbsp chia seeds
1 tbsp cornstarch
2 tsp instant coffee mix (or espresso powder)

1/2 tsp ground cinnamon

1/4 tsp salt

1/4 cup raw honey (or maple syrup)

2 cups low-fat chocolate milk

50 grams dark chocolate (at least 70%), finely chopped

1 tsp vanilla extract

Directions:

1. In a saucepan, mix together the chia seeds, cornstarch, coffee, cinnamon, and salt.
2. Over medium heat, add the raw honey and chocolate milk. Stir and cook for 5 minutes, stirring often until the mixture thickens.
3. Remove the mixture from the heat.
4. Add the dark chocolate and vanilla, whisking fast to prevent lumps.
5. Serve immediately. (Alternatively, you can put the mixture in a glass bowl. Cover it with plastic wrap directly on the surface and refrigerate for up to 5 days.)

#4   Banana Quesadillas

Ingredients:

1 whole wheat tortilla

1 large, very ripe banana

1 tbsp peanut butter

dark chocolate shavings (at least 70%, optional)

Directions:

1. Mash the banana in a bowl with a fork.
2. Get a tortilla wrap and spread peanut butter and the mashed banana on it.
3. Add dark chocolate shavings.
4. Fold or roll the tortilla.
5. Warm in the microwave for about 20 seconds. Slice and serve.

#5   Mango & Coconut Treat

Ingredients:

1 mango, cut into wedges

1 tbsp dry, shredded coconut

Directions:

1. Turn your oven to 'broil' and then position a rack in the upper third part of the oven.

2. Line a baking tray with foil or parchment paper.
3. Spread the dry, shredded coconut on a plate.
4. Dip each mango slice into the shredded coconut, pressing each to fully cover.
5. Arrange the mango slices in a single layer in the prepared pan and broil until the shredded coconut is nicely brown and slightly crispy.

#6   Sesame & Raisin Bombs

Ingredients:

1/3 cup honey (or maple syrup)

1/3 cup peanut butter

3/4 cup nonfat dry milk

3/4 cup sesame seeds

1/4 cup raisins

1/4 cup shredded coconut

Directions:

1. Place the shredded coconut on a plate. Set aside.
2. In a large bowl, thoroughly mix together the rest of the above ingredients.
3. Using a small ice cream scooper (or a 1 tbsp measuring spoon), scoop out some mixture and roll into balls using your hands.
4. Dip each ball into the shredded coconut.
5. Place in the refrigerator for at least 4 hours before enjoying them.

#7   No-Bake Chocolate Cookie

Ingredients:

1.5 cups raw almonds

1.5 cups dates, un-pitted

1/4 cup cacao powder

1/2 tsp pure vanilla extract

1/4 tsp sea salt

Filling:

8 oz almond milk cream cheese

5 tbsp maple syrup

1/2 tsp pure vanilla extract

Directions:

1. For the cookies: combine all the cookie ingredients into a food processor, and then process until everything comes together.

2. For the filling: Set up your stand mixer using the paddle attachment. Add all the filling ingredients and whip until very smooth.
3. **Roll out the cookie 'dough' between two pieces of parchment paper until it's about 1/4 inch thick.**
4. Using a round cookie cutter, cut out cookie rounds and put them on a wide platter (or cookie sheet)
5. Place the cookies in the refrigerator and chill for at least 30 minutes.
6. Take the chilled cookies out.
7. Place a half spoonful of cream cheese filling on one cookie and then top this off with another cookie round.
8. Press slightly so that the cream cheese filling spreads out evenly inside the cookie.
9. Eat right away or store the no-bake cookies in an airtight container in the refrigerator. They can last up to 7 days.

#8   Grapefruit Mango Sorbet

Ingredients:

1/4 cup water
2 tbsp cup cane sugar or coconut sugar
1/4 tsp ground ginger
1 large grapefruit, cut into segments
2 small scoops of mango sorbet
fresh mint (optional)

Directions:

1. In a small saucepan, simmer the water, cane sugar, and ginger for about 5 minutes or until the mixture is reduced to a thick syrup.
2. Divide the grapefruit segments over two dessert bowls.
3. Pour the ginger syrup over grapefruit and top with each with a scoop of mango sorbet and fresh mint.

#9   Coconut Ice Cream

Ingredients:

2 cans thick, full-fat coconut milk
2 cup heavy cream
1/4 cup coconut sugar
1 tsp. pure vanilla extract
Pinch kosher salt

Directions:

1. Chill the coconut milk in the refrigerator overnight.
2. Open the coconut milk cans, and then spoon out the solidified coconut cream at the top. Using a hand mixer, whip the coconut cream until creamy. Set aside.
3. In another bowl, using the hand mixer again, whip the heavy cream until soft peaks form.
4. Add in the rest of the coconut milk, coconut sugar, and vanilla.
5. Fold in the whipped coconut cream.
6. Transfer the mixture into a loaf pan and freeze overnight.

#10 Healthy Popcorn

Ingredients:

2 tbsp coconut oil

1/2 cup popcorn kernels, unsweetened and unbuttered

Directions:

1. Put a heavy-bottomed pot or pan over medium heat.
2. Add the coconut oil and wait until it's melted.
3. Take the pot off the heat. Add the popcorn kernels, cover the pot, and give it a quick shake to distribute the popcorn kernels inside it.
4. Set the pot back on the stove burner and wait for the tell-tale popping sounds. Shake the pot every now and then to ensure that the heat is reaching all the kernels.
5. Continue cooking until the popping sounds slow down to just about one pop per few seconds.
6. Take off the lid and place the popcorn in a big bowl. You can sprinkle the popcorn with a bit of salt or smoked paprika.

#11 Veggie Platter with Homemade Hummus

Ingredients:

1 cucumber

1 carrot

3 celery stalks

1 red bell pepper

1 green bell pepper

1 cup cauliflower florets

For the hummus:

1 can chickpeas, drained but reserve the liquid

1/4 cup tahini

1 tbsp lemon juice

1 tbsp extra-virgin olive oil

1 clove garlic, grated

1/4 tsp ground cumin

Salt and pepper to taste

Directions:

1. Slice all the vegetables, except the cauliflower, into sticks or whichever way you like them. (Note: Feel free to add any other vegetable you like too such as cherry tomatoes, olives, radishes, etc.) Arrange the vegetables on a big platter.

2. To make the hummus, put all the ingredients in a food processor and blend until you reach your desired consistency. Adjust the seasoning if necessary.

3. If the dip is too thick, add some water (or the drained chickpea water) a tablespoon at a time.

Bonus Recipes!

#1 Cauliflower Rice

Ingredients:

1 medium head cauliflower, cut into florets

1/2 tbsp garlic powder

1/2 tbsp turmeric powder

Salt and pepper to taste

Directions:

1. Heat the oven to 200°C.

2. Put the cauliflower florets into a food processor and 'pulse' until the cauliflower resembles rice granules.

3. Spread the cauliflower rice onto a large baking tray.

4. Add the garlic powder, turmeric powder, salt, and pepper. Mix to combine.

5. Bake the cauliflower rice for 20-25 mins, mixing halfway through.

#2 REAL Chicken Nuggets

Ingredients:

4 pieces, boneless, skinless chicken thighs

1 cup buttermilk

1/2 tbsp garlic powder

1/2 tbsp onion powder

1/2 tbsp dried thyme

Salt and pepper to taste

1 egg

1 cup whole-wheat breadcrumbs

1/2 cup dried shredded coconut

Directions:

1. Cut the chicken thighs into nugget-size pieces.
2. In a bowl, mix together the buttermilk and half of the garlic powder, onion powder, and dried thyme.
3. Place the chicken in the buttermilk mixture and refrigerate for at least 30 minutes. (Overnight is better.)
4. Preheat the oven to 180°C.
5. Lightly spray a baking sheet with cooking spray.
6. Take the chicken out and drain from the buttermilk marinade.
7. Lightly toast the whole wheat bread crumbs and shredded coconut.
8. Place the bread crumbs and coconut on a shallow plate to cool. Once cooled, add the remainder of your seasonings to the plate.
9. In a separate small bowl, lightly beat the egg.
10. Dip each nugget into the egg mixture, then onto the breadcrumb mixture. Press to thoroughly coat the chicken.
11. Place the nugget on the baking tray and do the same for all chicken pieces.
12. Bake for about 10 minutes.
13. Flip each nugget and bake for another 5 minutes or until the internal temperature of the chicken reaches 74°C.

#3   Baked Sweet Potato Wedges

Ingredients:

2 medium sweet potatoes

1/2 cup extra-virgin olive oil

Salt and pepper to taste

2 tbsp rosemary, finely chopped

Directions:

1. Preheat the oven to 200°C.
2. Wash and brush the sweet potatoes to get rid of any dirt.
3. Slice the sweet potatoes into wedges, and then place them in a shallow bowl.
4. Add the extra-virgin olive oil, rosemary, salt, and pepper. Toss to combine.
5. Place the wedges on a baking sheet and bake for 30-35 minutes.

#4   Avocado Chips

Ingredients:

1 large ripe avocado

1/2 cup Parmesan, grated

1 tsp lemon juice

1/2 tsp garlic powder

1/4 tsp dried oregano

Salt and pepper to taste

Directions:

1.   Preheat the oven to 175°C.

2.   Lightly spray two large baking sheets with cooking spray or line them with parchment paper.

3.   In a bowl, mash the avocado with a fork.

4.   Add the grated Parmesan, lemon juice, garlic powder, dried oregano, salt, and pepper to the avocado mash.

5.   Using a small ice cream scooper or a measuring spoon, scoop out a tablespoon of the mixture to the baking sheet. Leave space around each scoop, about 3 inches.

6.   Using the back of a wet spoon, spread and flatten the mixture thinly.

7.   Bake the 'chips' for around 30 minutes, or until crisp and golden.

8.   Cool and serve.

#5   Whole Wheat Banana Loaf

Ingredients:

1/3 cup coconut oil, melted

1/2 cup raw honey (or maple syrup)

2 large eggs

1/4 cup water, filtered

2 large very ripe bananas

1 tsp vanilla extract

1/4 tsp salt

1/2 tsp cinnamon

1.5 cups whole wheat flour

1 tsp baking soda

Directions:

1.   Preheat the oven to 165°C.

2.   Lightly grease a 9×5 inch loaf pan.

3. In a big bowl, whisk together the coconut oil and raw honey. Add the eggs and water. Mix well to combine.

4. Peel and mash the bananas.

5. In a separate bowl, mix together the bananas, vanilla, salt, and cinnamon.

6. Add the banana mixture to the wet ingredients. Stir to combine.

7. Whisk the whole wheat flour and baking soda together. Add this to the rest of the ingredients. Stir just to combine.

8. Place the batter into the greased loaf pan.

9. Bake for 55-65 minutes. To test if the banana loaf is done, insert a toothpick in the middle of the bread and take it out after a few seconds. If it comes out clean (i.e., hardly any crumbs are attached to it), the bread is done.

10. Cool the banana loaf for about 5 minutes. Remove from the loaf pan and move to a wire rack to cool for another half hour before slicing and serving.

Zero Sugar, Low-Carb Friendly Drinks

Apart from water, is there anything else you can drink? Yes, plenty! Following are some options for you. Of course, it goes without saying that the following drinks should be consumed as is, which means no adding of any sugar or sweetener whatsoever.

1. **Herbal tea.**

    Open yourself to the widely varied world of tea! Tea flavors range from light floral blends to deep and warm earthy flavors so there's a wide assortment to choose from. You can have it hot or cold too. Best of all, tea contains no sugar!

    Tea also offers A LOT of health benefits depending on the ingredient you use. For instance, chamomile tea is known to heal sinus issues and even migraines. Mint tea improves digestion and oral health. Ginger tea is great against sore throats and is known to boost the body's immune system. Rooibos tea, an herbal tea from South Africa, is believed to help with weight loss.

    Healthy example: Natural Chamomile Flower Tea

    Boil about a liter of water in a kettle or water boiler. Pinch off about 3-4 tablespoons worth of chamomile flowers direct from its stems. Put the boiled water into a teapot and let the chamomile flowers infuse in it for about 5 minutes. Drink and enjoy. (You can add a sprig of peppermint or a whole cinnamon stick in the pot too as well.)

2. **Lemon- or lime-infused water.**

    Who says you should only have this at fancy restaurants? Get yourself a nice, tall glass pitcher, fill it with filtered water and add a whole lemon or lime (or both!) cut into thin slices. Sip this hydrating, sugar-free drink throughout the day and see your skin improve too.

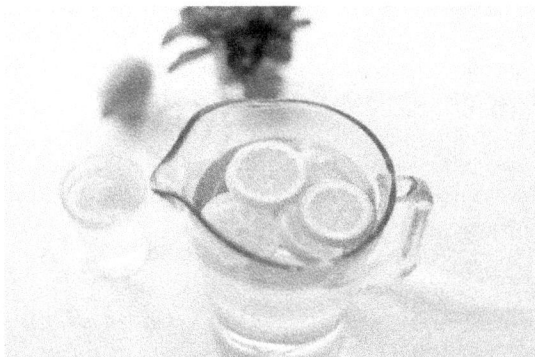

3. **Fruit- or herb-infused water.**
There's no need to confine yourself to citrus fruits. Flavor your water with fruit and/or herbs as well. The only thing with this option is that they may need some time. You can pretty much drink brewed teas and lemon/lime water immediately. Fruit and herbs, however, need a few hours to steep before they can really impart their flavors to the water.

Healthy example: Watermelon and Mint Water
Cut up some watermelon into chunks and put them in a pitcher. (Alternatively, you can use an infusion water bottle for on-the-go drinking.) Get some mint leaves and bruise them using the back of a knife. Add the mint to the watermelon and top it all off with filtered water. Set this in the fridge to cool for 4-5 hours.

4. **Flavored or unflavored sparkling water.**
Many people trying to quit sugar find it extremely hard to switch to plain water because of their HIGH consumption of soda drinks. The answer to that is sparkling water. Start with the flavored variety like peach mango, strawberry, cranberry, etc., and then gradually graduate to plain carbonated water. Before you know it, you'll be ready to switch to plain water in no time.

5. **Coffee!**
Skip the 1,000 calorie Frappuccino and go back to basics – have plain, unadulterated black coffee. Drip it, cold brew it, ice it, French press it. It doesn't matter. The rule of thumb is to have coffee as 'pure' as possible.

If you can't bear to switch to 'plain black' just yet, then add cinnamon or nutmeg to your cup. Just not sugar! You may also want to try changing coffee brands or testing other coffee flavors.

As your eating lifestyle changes, so will your taste buds. So don't be surprised that you find your coffee tasting 'different' now. It may not be just the lack of sugar.

I would of course suggest that you stick to just plain water or any of the zero sugar alternatives above from here on out. But if you do find yourself wanting just a tiny bit of sugary taste in your drinks, then I recommend the following.

6.   **Freshly-squeezed lemonade.**
Lemonade brings memories of lazy summer days and sticky fingers. Bring back the fun without the added sugar by making a simple syrup from healthy sweetener options like cane sugar, coconut sugar, raw honey, or agave nectar.
Boil a cup of water on the stove, and then add a cup of your healthy sweetener of choice. Stir to dissolve the sweetener and then remove the syrup from the heat. Juice a cup of lemon juice into a pitcher. Add 3 cups of filtered water and then add HALF of the simple syrup. Serve chilled with ice and fresh lemon slices.

7.   **Coconut water.**
Did you know that coconut water has low sugar content? With just 8-10 grams of sugar per cup, it's a great and refreshing alternative to water. It has many health benefits too.

Coconut water may lower blood sugar levels, help prevent the formation of kidney stones, has antioxidant properties, and is a great source of calcium and potassium.

8.   **Kombucha.**
Kombucha has been making waves in the health and wellness niche. And while its slightly sweet, slightly sour flavor is not for everyone, it's believed to have probiotic qualities which are great for gut health.

9.   **Plant-based milk.**
Cow's milk is not recommended while on a zero sugar diet because it contains natural sugar. Of course, that's still better than ADDED SUGAR but why not try plant-based milk instead such as almond milk, macadamia nut milk, or even flaxseed milk. Of course, go for the unsweetened versions of these milk alternatives.

Can you JUICE on a zero sugar diet?

It really depends on the *juice ingredients*. When people think of 'juicing', it's all about fruits. That's not good if you're on a zero sugar diet because fruits are high in natural sugars. What you should do, if you really want to juice, is to juice a healthy mix of fruits AND vegetables. Here are some juicing recipes you can try.

The Salad Juice
1 head romaine lettuce
1 handful of spinach
1 celery stalk
3 kale leaves
1 lemon, peeled
1-inch knob of fresh ginger

The 'Hulk'
1/2 green apple
3 kale leaves
8 mint
3 limes, peeled
1 cucumber
1 handful of spinach

Blackberry Green Juice
1/2 cup fresh blackberries
1/2 green apple
1 lemon, peeled
3 kale leaves
1/2 cup broccoli
1/2 cup fresh watercress
1/2 small cucumber

The Gut Health Juice
1 fennel stalk
1 celery stalk
1-inch knob of fresh ginger
1 big carrot
3 kale leaves
1/2 small cucumber
1 lemon, peeled

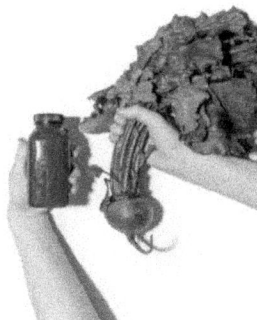

Beet It

1 small red beet

1 small carrot

1-inch knob of fresh ginger

1 lemon, peeled

2 handfuls spinach

1 celery stalk

The directions for the above juice options are the same: wash the ingredients thoroughly. If applicable, peel the produce. Put all the ingredients through a juicer and enjoy!

Note that it's best to drink fresh juice within 24 hours. Anything longer and the juice will start to lose some of its nutritional benefits.

Chapter 8

Improve Your Health Inside and Out

There's no doubt about it. Adapting a zero sugar, low carbohydrate eating lifestyle will do WONDERS for your health. And as you start your healthy living journey, I do recommend that you stick to making dietary changes first.

You see, the reason many people fail with their weight loss and/or healthy living efforts is that they take on too many things too soon.

So I say – focus on healthy eating first.

Once you see the amazing results that healthy eating brings, go ahead and take further steps regarding your health and fitness levels.

Trust me – you WILL want to do more than just eat healthy once you start losing weight and feeling more energetic.

But once you reach that stage, what do you do? That moment is the perfect time to address your **mental health** and **physical fitness** levels.

Mental - Mindset Changes Toward Food

Life throws A LOT of curveballs. You know this. You're bound to encounter certain life events (e.g., birthday parties, Holiday dinners, work-related celebrations, etc.) that may make you stumble with your healthy eating, healthy living habits.

And that's OK!

Here are a few mindset changes you may need to adapt to help you positively move on if ever you go 'off track'.

1. Food is NOT your enemy.

   Here's the truth – food was never your enemy. In the beginning, your *food choices* may have been your undoing. However, as we discussed in Chapter 2, sugar is addictive. So, in many ways, you were compelled to make unhealthy food choices later on.

So, here's the mindset change you need to adapt – stop thinking of unhealthy food as the enemy you need to defeat.

In fact, go ahead and enjoy unhealthy foods **once in a while**, and **in moderation**.

2. Food is not a measure of yourself as a human being. Food does not define you. Many people undergoing dietary changes feel that if they slip and eat unhealthy food, they somehow fail as a person. This is not a healthy mindset to have.

Food is there to nourish your body; to give you the right energy so that you can live life to the fullest. It should not define you as a person.

Instead, I suggest you list down all your GOOD qualities. If you lost your way while you were leading an unhealthy life, it's time to get to know yourself again!

Listing down your positive qualities will not only boost your mood but will also remind you that you're MORE than your food choices.

Often, when someone is asked to write down what they like or what's good about themselves they don't want to do it because they think it's being vain. Not at all! It's ALWAYS better to be positive than to be negative about yourself.

Another obstacle is that people often don't know WHAT to list down about themselves. Well, let me help you.

Following are a few questions I encourage you to answer now.

- What do you like about yourself?
- What positive characteristics do you have?
- What are some of your achievements?
- What are some challenges (big or small) that you've overcome?
- What talents or skills do you have?

Are you still finding it hard to say something great about yourself? Here's another question.

What has a friend done for you lately?
Sample answer: She cooked and sent me some soup when I was not feeling well.

Now, ask yourself this: would I do **something like that for a friend who's sick?**

If you say yes, then you can list down the following positive qualities for yourself.

- I am a great friend.
- I have empathy.
- I'm someone people can count on.

3.   Think and consider before you eat something.
Every time you're faced with an unhealthy food item, take a few seconds and ask yourself – *is this worth it?*

If it's not, let it go and move on to a healthier alternative.
If it is, go ahead and enjoy it.
If it's not and you eat it anyway, enjoy it, and then get back on track tomorrow.

That's it. Move on.

The point is that you shouldn't dwell on it. Contemplating it over and over simply makes it a big issue in your mind when in reality it isn't or it doesn't have to be!

4.   Willpower has nothing to do with your zero sugar journey.
Willpower is the ability to fight short-term temptation in favor of long-term goals. But instead of trying to practice 'willpower' every single day, why not just make a slight modification in your mindset and character?

For example, why not say "I will only eat chips on weekends; Saturday or Sunday night only."

All of a sudden you removed any feelings of deprivation and instead made a decision to eat chips only on weekends. The *pressure* of trying to avoid chips Monday to Friday is gone because you've delegated the decision to the weekend.

Try it now. Close your eyes, take a deep breath, and think of ONE trigger food with which you struggle. Open your eyes, let your breath out, and state your rules.

Examples:

- I will eat one slice of chocolate cake, but only during birthday parties. (So if there's no chocolate cake at the next birthday party you attend, no cake for you.)

- I will drink one alcoholic beverage during parties, but only if I'm with Tina. (So, if Tina's not with you, you don't drink alcohol.)

5. Let go of shame.

Did you know that shame can be a negative, and paralyzing emotion?[38]

Ok, so you indulged in some deep-fried chicken, pasta carbonara, a slice of cake, and a few glasses of wine last night.

Many people on a health or weight loss journey would wake up feeling ashamed by this. But it's not the food that may prove to be your undoing. It's the feeling of shame that you associate with it.

Shame can be a self-defeating emotion that if you give in to it – you may end up giving up what you've accomplished altogether. (This is the 'if I can't stick to my plan, then I better give up' mentality)

So, here's the mindset shift you need to make – accept that you gave in, take responsibility for it, and then get back directly on your healthy lifestyle routine.

6. Healthy eating is SELF-LOVE.

Many people think that switching to a healthier eating pattern is all about deprivation. That it's a punishment to eat healthily. They're wrong.

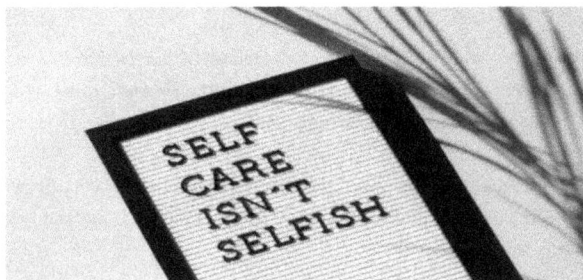

Healthy eating is practicing self-care and self-love.

Do you want to age gracefully? Do you want to look older, or younger than your real age? Do you want to be out of breath all the time and have difficulty moving, or do you want to be flexible and energetic now and in the years to come?

Do you see it? Choosing to eat healthy means you love yourself because you want to live a long and happy life.

7.   Keep moving forward.

You're losing weight and feeling great – good for you! Don't stop now. Keep moving forward!

Learn and educate yourself more about food, your body, and what you like and dislike about health and well-being in general.

For instance, many people on a zero sugar, low carbohydrate diet find themselves learning about a new world of ingredients. So perhaps now would be a good time to travel and deepen your knowledge about a specific food ingredient (e.g., travel to India to know about different spices).

Don't want to travel? Then how about just taking an online course about meal prepping, or cooking more vegetarian dishes?

Truly, the world is your oyster.

Physical - Move Your Way to Fitness

One of the ways to move forward and build on your healthy eating, healthy living success is to **GET PHYSICAL.** Yes, we're talking about movement, being more physically active, exercising!

If you want to lose weight and be healthier, then yes, changing your eating lifestyle is enough to melt the pounds. However, if you want to tone your body and improve your fitness levels, then you need to move.

Besides, what are you going to do with all the EXTRA ENERGY you have after following my 7-Day Zero-Sugar Diet Plan?

And in case you're still on the edge about WHY you should exercise, let the following facts persuade you.

1. Exercise FIGHTS sickness and diseases. Physical activity improves your body's high-density lipoprotein (HDL) cholesterol levels while lowering unhealthy triglycerides in your body. This health combo drastically lowers your risk of contracting cardiovascular illnesses.

   Consistent exercise helps prevent many health issues such as stroke, metabolic syndrome, high blood pressure, type 2 diabetes, different types of cancer, arthritis, and others.

   Exercise also boosts cognitive function, improving memory and thinking functions.

2. Exercise improves your mood. Exercise releases *endorphins*, chemicals that relate with receptors in your brain to lower pain perception. It also stimulates chemicals that can make you feel happier, less stressed, and more relaxed. So if you ever need an emotional lift, get moving!
   Regular exercise also improves your physical appearance, which in turn can boost your self-confidence and self-esteem.

3. Exercise gives you even more energy. Regular exercise improves muscle strength and advances your physical endurance. This is because physical activity delivers oxygen and nutrients to body tissues and helps your cardiovascular system work better. As a result, you'll have more energy to do daily tasks and chores.

4. Exercise supports quality sleep. Yes, you'll feel tired after an exercise session but in a GOOD way. As such, it can help you sleep faster and experience better quality sleep. However, don't exercise strenuously just before bedtime as this may leave you too energized to sleep. If you want to use exercise for the purpose of winding down, then a light, meditative yoga session is ideal.

5. Exercise boosts 'bedroom activity'. If you lack energy and have a negative body image of yourself as a result of being overweight, it's understandable that intimacy in the bedroom takes a backseat.
   The good news is that with consistent exercise, you can increase energy levels and your self-confidence, which in turn can revive your sex life.

   But it's not just about having more energy. Exercise itself enhances arousal in women because it increases and sustains levels of an enzyme that boosts genital blood flow and arousal.

6. Exercise supports long-term, permanent weight loss.[39] Regular exercise helps maintain weight loss and prevent future weight gain. This is because exercise helps the body burn calories. The more strenuous the exercise routine, the more calories are burned.

    However, note that you DO NOT need a fancy gym membership to establish an effective exercise routine.

    No equipment workouts: take the stairs instead of the elevator at work, run outdoors, engage in bodyweight exercises, dance, and more!

    When possible, invest in inexpensive equipment like a pair of dumbbells, a gym ball, elastic bands, or even a hula hoop!

    Do remember though that **consistency is key**. Keep moving to keep burning calories.

7. Exercise can open a whole new social network for you! Believe it or not, exercising can lead to new friends. For example, early morning walks or jogs can reveal others in your neighborhood who have the same routine. Start with a smile, nod, or wave as a greeting. Next time, strike up a short and easy conversation. Who knows where that will lead?

    If you're attending local exercise classes at your local gym, great! You already have a group of people interested in the same thing as you are. Again, don't be afraid to start a short and easy conversation with someone. Everything starts with 'hello'.

So, how much physical activity do you need?
According to the U.S. Department of Health and Human Services, adults should engage in a combination of aerobic and strength activities each week.[40]

Aerobic exercises are any activities that promote cardiovascular conditioning. Anything that requires a bit of effort and gets your heart rate up will do.

Following is what's recommended for aerobic activities.

> ➤ Do at least 2.5 hours of light to moderate aerobic activity, or 75 minutes of energetic aerobic activity each week. A combination of light and dynamic aerobic activity is ok too.

> ➢ Spread out your exercise times over the week. That is, it's better for your heart and your overall condition to do 30 minutes of aerobic activity per day than exercising for 2 full hours on a weekend.

> ➢ For greater health benefits and to assist with weight loss success and maintenance, a minimum of 300 minutes (1 hour a day, 5 days) is recommended.

Strength training, also known as weight training or resistance training, builds muscle endurance and thus makes your body stronger.

Following is what's recommended for strength training.

> ➢ Perform strength training exercises targeting all major muscle groups at least twice a week.

> ➢ Try to perform at least one set of every strength training exercise using a resistance level that's hard enough to tire your muscles. (One step is equivalent to about 12-15 repetitions.)

Sample 14-Day Fitness Routine for Beginners

If you're new to fitness activities, that's ok! No one expects you to burst out the front door, and participate in a half marathon. Slow but sure is the key. Remember, **everyone starts at Level 1.**

The outline below is a simple fitness guide for beginners. Try and do the aerobic exercise for at least 30 minutes each day. If you can't do that, start at 15 minutes each day and work your way up.

Notice that the strength training exercises are not introduced until the following week. If you feel fit and have the time to incorporate them on Day 1, great! If not, that's ok too.

What's important is this – START!

Day	Aerobic Exercise	Strength Training Exercise
Day 1	Brisk walking*	
Day 2	Power walking**	

Day 3	Brisk walking	
Day 4	Power walking	
Day 5	Brisk walking	
Day 6	Power walking	
Day 7	Brisk walking + Light jog***	
Day 8	Brisk walking + Light jog	Bodyweight squats[a]
Day 9	Power walking + Light jog***	Beginner plank[b]
Day 10	Power walking + Light jog	Bodyweight squats
Day 11	Brisk walking	Beginner plank
Day 12	Power walking	Bodyweight squats
Day 13	Brisk walking + Light jog****	Beginner plank
Day 14	Light jog	Full plank

Fitness Notes:

* **Brisk walking** – just walk a little bit faster than your CURRENT walking speed. The goal is simply to be a little bit out of breath, but nothing that you cannot manage for 15-30 minutes straight.

** **Power walking** –walk a little bit faster than your brisk walking pace. Add some PROPER arm swinging if you can. How? Bend your elbows at 90 degrees. Don't clench your hands, relax them. Keep your elbows close to your body, and let them naturally swing back and forth as you walk.

*** **Brisk/Power walking + Light jog** – Brisk walk or power walk, and then light jog at intervals. For example, brisk walk for 10 minutes, and then lightly jog for 1 minute. When this gets easy, brisk walk for 10 minutes and then lightly jog for 3 minutes. Keep on going and increasing the light jogging minutes as your aerobic endurance improves.

The end goal is to be able to lightly jog for 15 or 30 minutes straight.

Other light aerobic exercise ideas: swimming, biking, cycling, dancing, etc.
As for strength training exercises, I suggest you do them immediately after your aerobic exercises. Your muscles are all warmed up at this stage, so it's best to do them now.

If time does not permit that, then make sure you do some warm-up exercises for at least 5 minutes before squatting or planking.

[a] **Bodyweight squats** are one of the easiest resistance exercises you can do. Simply stand straight with your feet hip-width apart. Tighten your stomach muscles, and then start lowering yourself down as if you're going to sit on a chair. Pause and then stand back up. Repeat the movement until you do 12-15 repetitions.

[b] **Beginner planks** are not only easy to do anytime, anywhere; they also target A LOT of muscles in the body so it's a great weight training activity.

The image below is for a full plank, which is the goal

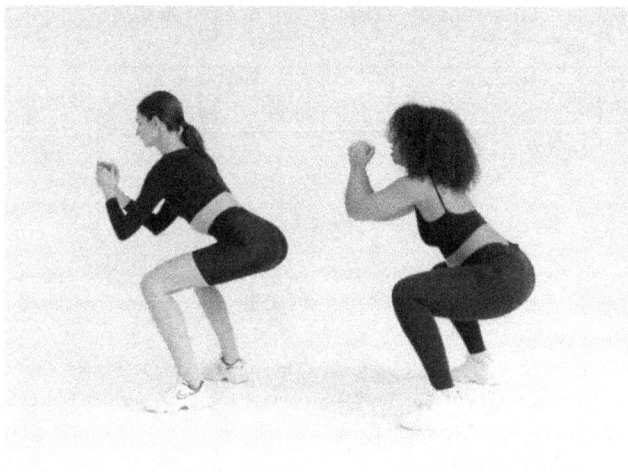

For a beginner plank, bring your knees to the floor and extend your arms (i.e., don't bend your elbow). Hold the pose for 5 seconds. If you can do it longer, great! If not just build upon that time, going from 5 seconds to 10 seconds, to 15 seconds, and so on.

Once you hit 60 seconds, move on to do a full plank and build the time you can hold that pose until you reach 60 seconds.

From there, you can do dozens of plank variations such as side planks, plank jacks, up and down planks, side tap planks, body saw planks, and much more.

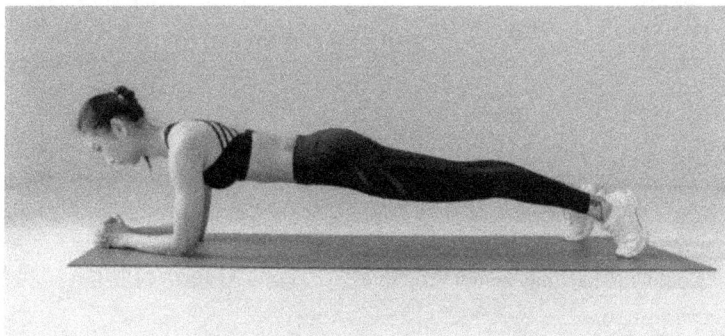

Other beginner strength training exercise ideas: walking lunges, bear crawl, dumbbell rows, etc.

Leave a 1-click review!

Customer Reviews

★★★★★ 2

5.0 out of 5 stars ▾

5 star		100%
4 star		0%
3 star		0%
2 star		0%
1 star		0%

See all verified purchase reviews ›

Share your thoughts with other customers

Write a customer review

I would be incredibly grateful if you take just 60 seconds to write just a brief review on Amazon, even if it's just a few sentences.

https://www.amazon.com/review/create-review-asin=B09MHF2XQ1

Conclusion

I t's great you decided to prioritize and take care of yourself and I thank you for selecting the Healthy Eating for Healthy Living guide as your health journey partner.

Author Thomas Sterner said **"Everything in life worth achieving requires practice"**, and that is definitely true for anyone embarking on a zero sugar, low carbohydrate eating lifestyle.

Your attempts at kicking sugar and its harmful effects on your life may be tough and frustrating at times but I assure you – if you follow what I outlined in this eBook, and keep on practicing these strategies, **YOU WILL SUCCEED.**

I know because as I mentioned at the start, I was just like you.

I was feeling miserable, not liking the way I was looking, letting myself and people around me down, and worst of all, **I was truly starting to believe that I couldn't change anything – UNTIL I DID.**

Today, I got up bursting with energy and excited about the day ahead. I look forward to what I need to do, knowing that I'm more than physically able to do them.

I'm mentally and emotionally stable and love the woman I see looking right back at me in the mirror.

And it all starts with KNOWLEDGE.

In this eBook, you learned that:

> - Sweet, sugary foods are not feel-good friends. They're health adversaries that diminish the quality of life.
> - Sugar addiction is REAL. However, just like any learned compulsion, you can unlearn it!
> - Adapting a zero sugar, low carbohydrate eating lifestyle gives you benefits beyond weight loss. You increase your body's ability to heal from sugar-related illnesses; you boost your energy levels; you sleep better; you improve your gut health; you lower your risk of contracting life-threatening diseases such as cancer; you improve brain function; you improve your emotional and mental state. And so much more!

> ➢ Success depends on the right preparation. To triumph with a zero sugar diet plan, it's important to set yourself up for success by doing things like clearing out your kitchen of unhealthy food items, learning mindful eating techniques, discovering non-food-related rewards, educating yourself on how to shop for healthy food, and so on.
> ➢ Living a healthy life is NOT about deprivation; it's about proper substitution.
> ➢ Meal planning and meal prepping can mean the difference between a healthy meal and an unhealthy one.
> ➢ Avoiding sugar is more than just paying attention to what you eat and drink. Your MIND plays a vital role in healing your sugar addiction.

And of course, thanks to the easy recipes in Chapter 7, you learned that healthy eating is not so difficult a change after all.

Truly, everything you need to lead a happier, healthier, and longer life is here. There's only one thing left to do - START.

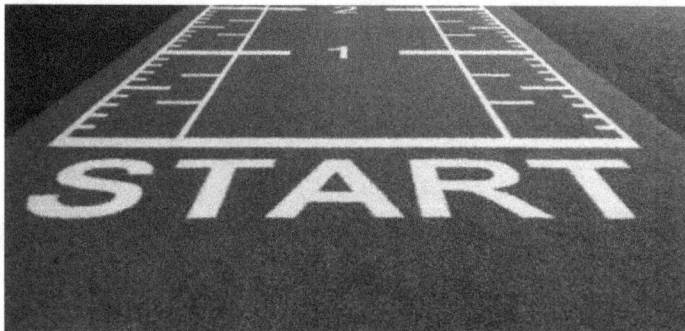

Note: If you found this eBook useful, do not forget to leave a review on Amazon to let others know how much you appreciated it. Thank you very much!

My other books you will love!

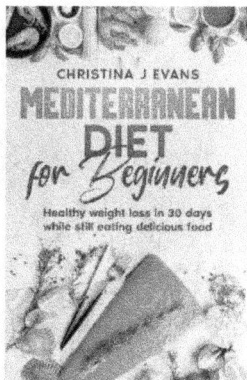

Amazon.com/dp/B09MJ5282Q

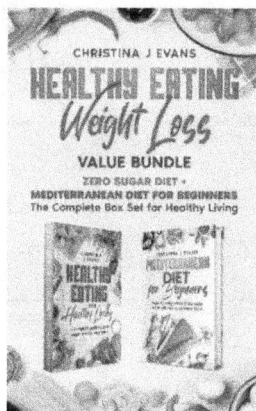

Amazon.com/dp/B09MHF2XQ1

Don't forget to grab your GIFT!!!

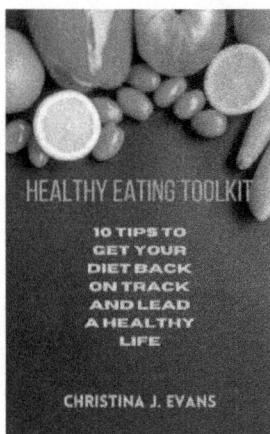

http://christinajevans.com/healthy-eating.pdf

Joining the HL Community

Looking to build your healthy eating lifestyle? If so, then check out the Healthy Living (HL) Community here:

www.facebook.com/groups/1004091000384321/

Appendices

Appendix A – A List of Grocery Staples and their Glycemic Load

A low glycemic load (GL) value keeps blood sugar levels consistent so that you don't experience that roller-coaster style of sugar highs and crashes. And since it's very important to regulate blood sugar levels for effective weight loss, the table below shows GL levels. As a general rule, the lower the GL value the better it is for a zero sugar, low carbohydrate diet.

ITEM	GLYCEMIC LOAD	SERVING SIZE
Vegetables		
Broccoli, cooked	0	78g (1/2 cup)
Cabbage, cooked	0	75g (1/2 cup)
Celery, raw	0	62g (1 stalk)
Cauliflower	0	100g (1 cup)
Green Beans	0	135g (1 cup)
Mushrooms	0	70g (1 cup)
Spinach	0	30g (1 cup)
Carrot, raw	1	15g (1 large)
Tomato	1.5	123g (1 med)
Peas, Frozen	3.4	72g (1/2 cup)
Beets, canned	9.6	246g (1/2 cup)
Parsnip	11.6	78g (1/2 cup)
Sweet Potato	12.4	133g (1 cup)
Yam	16.8	136g (1 cup)
Fruits		
Avocado	0	50g
Lime	1	120g
Strawberry	1	120g

Apricot	3	120g
Grapefruit	3	120g
Lemon	3	120g
Cantaloupe	4	120g
Guava	4	120g
Nectarines	4	120g
Oranges	4	120g
Pear	4	120g
Watermelon	4	120g
Blueberries	5	120g
Peach	5	120g
Plum	5	120g
Apple	6	120g
Pineapple	6	120g
Kiwi	7	120g
Mango	8	120g
Cherries	9	120g
Prunes	10	60g
Banana	11	120g
Grapes	11	120g
Oats		
Steel-cut oats		
Old-fashioned or whole oats		
Quick or instant oats (unflavored)		
Nuts (Raw, Unsalted/Unroasted)		
Almonds	0	30g (handful)
Walnuts	0	30g (handful)
Pistachios	0	30g (handful)
Peanuts	0	30g (handful)
Cashew	0	30g (handful)
Fats & Oils		

Extra Virgin Olive Oil		
Coconut oil		
Grass-fed butter		
Pasta, Breads, Rice		
Pasta/Bread: anything as long as they're whole-wheat or whole grain		
Rice: brown rice		
Canned Goods		
Canned tuna		
Canned salmon		
Meat/Protein		
Chicken	Eggs	
Beef	Lamb	
Fish	Pork	
Bacon (Go for the 'center cut'. The leaner the meat, the better.)		

Appendix B – The Most Common Sugar Names

One of the reasons it's so difficult to eliminate sugar from our diets is because they go by so many names! Following is a list of the most common sugar names today. Note that not all of the sugars listed below are bad per se. It's the amount of sugar that counts. As a rule of thumb, a total carbohydrate count of is 1–2 grams is still ok to consume in a low carbohydrate eating lifestyle.

Basic Simple Sugars (monosaccharides and disaccharides):	
1.	Dextrose
2.	Fructose
3.	Galactose
4.	Glucose
5.	Lactose
6.	Maltose

7.	Sucrose
	Solid or Granulated Sugars:
8.	Beet sugar
9.	Brown sugar
10.	Cane juice crystals
11.	Cane sugar
12.	Castor sugar
13.	Coconut sugar
14.	Confectioner's sugar (aka, powdered sugar)
15.	Corn syrup solids
16.	Crystalline fructose
17.	Date sugar
18.	Demerara sugar
19.	Dextrin
20.	Diastatic malt
21.	Ethyl maltol
22.	Florida crystals
23.	Golden sugar
24.	Glucose syrup solids
25.	Grape sugar
26.	Icing sugar
27.	Maltodextrin
28.	Muscovado sugar
29.	Panela sugar
30.	Raw sugar

31.	Sugar (granulated or table)
32.	Sucanat
33.	Turbinado sugar
34.	Yellow sugar
	Liquid or Syrup Sugars:
35.	Agave Nectar/Syrup
36.	Barley malt
37.	Blackstrap molasses
38.	Brown rice syrup
39.	Buttered sugar/buttercream
40.	Caramel
41.	Carob syrup
42.	Corn syrup
43.	Evaporated cane juice
44.	Fruit juice
45.	Fruit juice concentrate
46.	Golden syrup
47.	High-Fructose Corn Syrup (HFCS)
48.	Honey
49.	Invert sugar
50.	Malt syrup
51.	Maple syrup
52.	Molasses
53.	Rice syrup
54.	Refiner's syrup

55.	Sorghum syrup
56.	Treacle

References

1. Centers for Disease Control and Prevention. (2021, September 27). *Heart disease facts*. Centers for Disease Control and Prevention. Retrieved October 1, 2021, from https://www.cdc.gov/heartdisease/facts.htm.

2. *2019 Philips World Sleep Day Survey Results - United States*. (n.d.). Retrieved October 1, 2021, from https://www.usa.philips.com/c-dam/b2c/master/experience/smartsleep/world-sleep-day/2019/2019-philips-world-sleep-day-survey-results.pdf.

3. Spiegel, K., Tasali, E., Penev, P., & Cauter, E. V. (2004). Brief communication: Sleep curtailment in healthy young men is associated with decreased leptin levels, elevated ghrelin levels, and increased hunger and appetite. *Annals of Internal Medicine, 141*(11), 846. https://doi.org/10.7326/0003-4819-141-11-200412070-00008

4. Breymeyer, K. L., Lampe, J. W., McGregor, B. A., & Neuhouser, M. L. (2016). Subjective mood and energy levels of healthy weight and overweight/obese healthy adults on high-and low-glycemic-load experimental diets. *Appetite, 107*, 253–259. https://doi.org/10.1016/j.appet.2016.08.008

5. Lim, S. Y., Kim, E. J., Kim, A., Lee, H. J., Choi, H. J., & Yang, S. J. (2016). Nutritional factors affecting mental health. *Clinical Nutrition Research, 5*(3), 143. https://doi.org/10.7762/cnr.2016.5.3.143

6. McClain, A. D., van den Bos, W., Matheson, D., Desai, M., McClure, S. M., & Robinson, T. N. (2013). Visual illusions and plate design: The effects of plate rim widths and rim coloring on perceived food portion size. *International Journal of Obesity, 38*(5), 657–662. https://doi.org/10.1038/ijo.2013.169

7. Hitti, M. (2008, July 8). *Weight loss study: Keeping a food diary helps shed extra pounds*. WebMD. Retrieved September 1, 2021, from https://www.webmd.com/diet/news/20080708/keeping-food-diary-helps-lose-weight.

8. Johnson, R. K., Appel, L. J., Brands, M., Howard, B. V., Lefevre, M., Lustig, R. H., Sacks, F., Steffen, L. M., & Wylie-Rosett, J. (2009). Dietary sugars intake and cardiovascular health. *Circulation, 120*(11), 1011–1020. https://doi.org/10.1161/circulationaha.109.192627

9. Avena, N. M., Rada, P., & Hoebel, B. G. (2008). Evidence for sugar addiction: Behavioral and neurochemical effects of intermittent, excessive sugar intake. *Neuroscience & Biobehavioral Reviews, 32*(1), 20–39. https://doi.org/10.1016/j.neubiorev.2007.04.019

10. Faruque, S., Tong, J., Lacmanovic, V., Agbonghae, C., Minaya, D., & Czaja, K. (2019). The dose makes the poison: Sugar and obesity in the United States – A

Review. *Polish Journal of Food and Nutrition Sciences*, 69(3), 219–233. https://doi.org/10.31883/pjfns/110735

11. Delli Bovi AP;Di Michele L;Laino G;Vajro P; (n.d.). *Obesity and obesity related diseases, sugar consumption and bad oral health: A fatal epidemic mixtures: The pediatric and odontologist point of View*. Translational medicine @ UniSa. Retrieved October 1, 2021, from https://pubmed.ncbi.nlm.nih.gov/28775964/.

12. R, O., B, G., & KR, U. (n.d.). *low carbohydrate Diet*. Europe PMC. Retrieved September 1, 2021, from https://europepmc.org/article/NBK/nbk537084.

13. Quagliani, D., & Felt-Gunderson, P. (2016). **Closing America's fiber intake gap.** *American Journal of Lifestyle Medicine*, 11(1), 80–85. https://doi.org/10.1177/1559827615588079

14. Harvey, C. J., Schofield, G. M., & Williden, M. (2018). The use of nutritional supplements to induce ketosis and reduce symptoms associated with keto-induction: A narrative review. *PeerJ*, 6. https://doi.org/10.7717/peerj.4488

15. B;, A. K. A.-S. E. A.-S. (n.d.). *The effect of tongue scraper on mutans streptococci and lactobacilli in patients with caries and periodontal disease*. Odonto-stomatologie tropicale = Tropical dental journal. Retrieved September 1, 2021, from https://pubmed.ncbi.nlm.nih.gov/16032940/.

16. *The link between taste buds, obesity, more*. Cornell Research. (2019, November 7). Retrieved September 2021, from https://research.cornell.edu/news-features/link-between-taste-buds-obesity-more.

17. *Losing weight, especially in the belly, improves sleep quality, according to a Johns Hopkins Study - 11/06/2012*. Johns Hopkins Medicine, based in Baltimore, Maryland. (n.d.). Retrieved September 2021, from https://www.hopkinsmedicine.org/news/media/releases/losing_weight_especia lly_in_the_belly_improves_sleep_quality_according_to_a_johns_hopkins_stu dy.

18. Rejeski, W. J., Ip, E. H., Bertoni, A. G., Bray, G. A., Evans, G., Gregg, E. W., & Zhang, Q. (2012). Lifestyle change and mobility in obese adults with type 2 diabetes. *New England Journal of Medicine*, 366(13), 1209–1217. https://doi.org/10.1056/nejmoa1110294

19. *Dealing With Feelings When You're Overweight*. Rady Children's Hospital-San Diego. (2014, September). Retrieved September 1, 2021, from https://www.rchsd.org/health-articles/dealing-with-feelings-when-youre-overweight/.

20. Burri, B. J. (2011). Evaluating Sweet Potato as an intervention food to prevent vitamin A deficiency. *Comprehensive Reviews in Food Science and Food Safety*, 10(2), 118–130. https://doi.org/10.1111/j.1541-4337.2010.00146.x

21. Matito, C., Agell, N., Sanchez-Tena, S., Torres, J. L., & Cascante, M. (2011). Protective effect of structurally diverse grape procyanidin fractions against UV-

induced cell damage and death. *Journal of Agricultural and Food Chemistry*, *59*(9), 4489–4495. https://doi.org/10.1021/jf103692a

22. Fat and salt combined is a toxic mix for our health and waistlines. (2016, March 10). Retrieved from https://www.deakin.edu.au/about-deakin/news-and-media-releases/articles/fat-and-salt-combined-is-a-toxic-mix-for-our-health-and-waistlines.

23. Fernstrom, J. D. (2007). Health issues relating to monosodium glutamate used in the Diet. *Reducing Salt in Foods*, 55–76. https://doi.org/10.1533/9781845693046.1.55

24. Kristeller, J. L., & Hallett, C. B. (1999). An exploratory study of a meditation-based intervention for binge eating disorder. *Journal of Health Psychology*, *4*(3), 357–363. https://doi.org/10.1177/135910539900400305

25. About the Author: Chris Dunne Marketing Executive at Tameday., & Tameday., M. E. at. (2019, May 3). *Do naps at work increase productivity?* Tameday. Retrieved September 2021, from https://www.tameday.com/do-naps-at-work-increase-productivity/.

26. Mayo Foundation for Medical Education and Research. (2020, August 18). *Exercise and stress: Get moving to manage stress*. Mayo Clinic. Retrieved October 26, 2021, from https://www.mayoclinic.org/healthy-lifestyle/stress-management/in-depth/exercise-and-stress/art-20044469.

27. Stenblom, E.-L., Egecioglu, E., Landin-Olsson, M., & Erlanson-Albertsson, C. (2015). Consumption of thylakoid-rich spinach extract reduces hunger, increases satiety, and reduces cravings for palatable food in overweight women. *Appetite*, *91*, 209–219. https://doi.org/10.1016/j.appet.2015.04.051

28. Belluz, J., & Zarracina, J. (2016, April 28). *Why you shouldn't exercise to lose weight, explained with 60+ studies*. Vox. Retrieved October 1, 2021, from https://www.vox.com/2016/4/28/11518804/weight-loss-exercise-myth-burn-calories.

29. Xu, A. J., Schwarz, N., & Wyer, R. S. (2015). Hunger promotes acquisition of nonfood objects. *Proceedings of the National Academy of Sciences*, *112*(9), 2688–2692. https://doi.org/10.1073/pnas.1417712112

30. Wansink, B., Hanks, A. S., & Kaipainen, K. (2016). Slim by design. *Health Education & Behavior*, *43*(5), 552–558. https://doi.org/10.1177/1090198115610571

31. Leidy, H. J., Clifton, P. M., Astrup, A., Wycherley, T. P., Westerterp-Plantenga, M. S., Luscombe-Marsh, N. D., Woods, S. C., & Mattes, R. D. (2015). The role of protein in weight loss and maintenance. *The American Journal of Clinical Nutrition*, *101*(6). https://doi.org/10.3945/ajcn.114.084038

32. Westerterp, K. R. (2004). Diet induced thermogenesis. *Nutrition & Metabolism*, *1*(1), 5. https://doi.org/10.1186/1743-7075-1-5

33. Dai, H., Milkman, K. L., & Riis, J. (2014). The fresh start effect: Temporal landmarks motivate aspirational behavior. *Management Science, 60*(10), 2563–2582. https://doi.org/10.1287/mnsc.2014.1901

34. Helander, E. E., Wansink, B., & Chieh, A. (2016). Weight gain over the holidays in three countries. *New England Journal of Medicine, 375*(12), 1200–1202. https://doi.org/10.1056/nejmc1602012

35. *Food Safety and Inspection Service.* Home | Food Safety and Inspection Service. (n.d.). Retrieved October 26, 2021, from https://www.fsis.usda.gov/.

36. Benedict, K., Jackson, B. R., Chiller, T., & Beer, K. D. (2018). Estimation of direct healthcare costs of fungal diseases in the United States. *Clinical Infectious Diseases, 68*(11), 1791–1797. https://doi.org/10.1093/cid/ciy776

37. Martins, N., Ferreira, I. C., Barros, L., Silva, S., & Henriques, M. (2014). Candidiasis: Predisposing factors, prevention, diagnosis and alternative treatment. *Mycopathologia, 177*(5-6), 223–240. https://doi.org/10.1007/s11046-014-9749-1

38. Sussex Publishers. (n.d.). *Overcoming the paralysis of toxic shame.* Psychology Today. Retrieved October 26, 2021, from https://www.psychologytoday.com/us/blog/overcoming-destructive-anger/201704/overcoming-the-paralysis-toxic-shame.

39. RIEBE, D., BLISSMER, B., GREENE, G., CALDWELL, M., RUGGIERO, L., STILLWELL, K., & NIGG, C. (2005). Long-term maintenance of exercise and healthy eating behaviors in overweight adults. *Preventive Medicine, 40*(6), 769–778. https://doi.org/10.1016/j.ypmed.2004.09.023

40. U.S. Department of Health and Human Services. (n.d.). Physical Activity Guidelines for Americans Summary - 2nd edition.

Mediterranean Diet for Beginners

Healthy weight loss in 30 days while still eating delicious food

By Christina J Evans

Just for You

A free gift to our readers

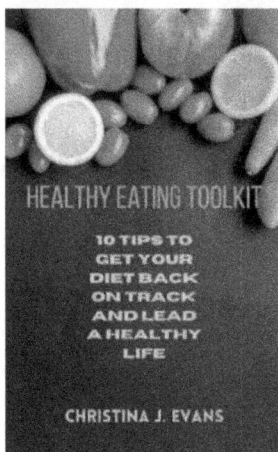

Click here

http://christinajevans.com/healthy-eating.pdf

Joining the HL Community

Looking to build your healthy eating lifestyle? If so, then check out the Healthy Living (HL) Community here:

www.facebook.com/groups/1004091000384321/

Introduction

I t is a general consensus that if you eat healthily, you will live a longer and more fulfilling life, but people find it really hard to stick with diets or with eating healthy because it asks you to make an effort which is not easy if you are living a fast-paced life. The people who do try to make an effort are unable to sustain it for more than 6 months simply because there is no pleasure in eating bland and tasteless food. If you are eating healthy, but your physical and mental health is still suffering, then is it worth it? This is why the Mediterranean diet is so different from other diets. It is not just a diet; it is a way of living.

Fast food has become a go-to meal because it's quick, cheap, and you don't have to put in an effort to eat it. A study conducted on childhood obesity proved that fast food was linked to a higher BMI (Body Mass Index) score, a higher body fat percentage, and a higher chance of obesity (K.Fraser, 2012). This is true because whether you believe it or not, food has a lot of control over how we feel, and eating fast food is not pleasurable. Research has also proven that eating fast food leads to depression or an increased risk of depression (Sánchez-Villegas, 2011). Of course, when you live a fast-paced life because you are constantly working and eating unfulfilling food that does not enrich your body, this results in a lifestyle that starts weighing on you over time.

"I have been on a diet for 2 weeks, and all I have lost is 14 days." – Totie Fields

I think we all have had times when we suddenly wake up one day and want to live a healthier lifestyle. Perhaps your health is declining due to the added weight, or you aren't as fit as you used to be. In any case, you want to try and live a healthier life so you can live for longer without increasing your risk of heart disease and high blood pressure. The problem is, losing weight is by no means an easy task, but sometimes, it is a necessity, and diets can be incredibly difficult, especially if you don't know the right way to go as there are many choices especially when you still want to be able to enjoy your meals.

I first started dieting because I was extremely conscious of my body weight and was insecure about my body fat. My immunity was lower because of my unhealthy eating habits, and I was getting sick more often. I decided to research healthy eating options not only because of my body weight but also to get healthier, especially since I know how hard it is to get out of eating unhealthy food once you get into it. While it may seem like changing your diet is a simple thing, people who have actually made the change or

attempted to make a change know how hard it really is, considering that your whole lifestyle now revolves around how, what, and where you eat.

Healthy Eating Weight Loss Value Bundle- Complete Box Set for Beginners

To be honest, I struggled a lot when I first started to diet. I couldn't really find a suitable diet plan, and when I found one, it felt like I was torturing myself because all the recipes were either really hard to recreate or bland and tasteless. I am a foodie, and there is no doubt that I love food, so when I started to diet, my primary goal was to create healthy food that wouldn't ask me to compromise on taste. That is when I started to get into the Mediterranean diet, which I knew would be best suited for my situation. It helps you lose weight and is also incredibly healthy for you since it uses a lot of fresh vegetables, herbs, nuts, and fish. In addition, the Mediterranean diet doesn't ask you to eliminate certain ingredients that are usually considered "bad," such as red meat. Instead, the diet lowers your consumption, which makes the diet a lot more enjoyable since you aren't compromising on your favorite foods.

The Mediterranean diet originated in the countries that border the Mediterranean Sea, and it is not a diet at all; rather, it is a way of life and a culinary tradition that focuses on using fresh vegetables and fruits with fresh protein. The diet uses local and sustainable ingredients to promote a natural and healthy life. There is a heavy focus on seafood and olive oil or olives in this diet, and that is because these ingredients are locally available in the region; hence they are "fresh." The premise of the diet itself is simple – eat whole foods that are in season and fresh and avoid processed foods with additives.

The Mediterranean diet has a lot of health benefits: it lowers the risk of cardiovascular disease because it contains a lot more minerals and vitamins than typical processed foods, there is also a correlation between the Mediterranean diet and a longer lifespan since the diet contains an abundance of nutrition and antioxidants which can fight the signs of aging, and most of all, the Mediterranean diet can help you lose and manage weight especially if you pair it with physical activity and lots of exercises.

We will be exploring topics on how you can switch to a sustainable healthy lifestyle which includes Mediterranean diets. I will provide a step-by-step guide that will help you make the switch to the Mediterranean diet much easier. The Mediterranean diet used to be based on the Mediterranean diet pyramid. In recent years, the U.S. guide to healthy eating has changed, which means that now the healthy way of eating includes half a plate of fruit and veggies while the other half should have protein, grains, and dairy. The U.S. guide is updated every 5 years, and currently, the core elements that make up a healthy diet are – all kinds of vegetables, fruits, grain, protein foods, and oils. We will discuss this in greater detail in the relevant chapters. (*Dietary Guide for Americans 2020-2025*,

2020). Aside from that, you will get to learn different culinary techniques and learn how to modify the diet to fit ingredients that might be available for you locally, and of course, you will find tons of new and delicious recipes.

If you have been struggling to adhere to a healthy way of eating and want to stress less about your health, the Mediterranean diet is the solution. It is not only easy and fast to prepare, but it is also inexpensive. And, if you want to live a life free of health issues without having to sacrifice flavor, then read on!

To your healthy living,

Christina J. Evans

Female Body Fat Expert | Healthy Living Advocate

Chapter 1

Understanding the Mediterranean Diet

The Mediterranean diet has been the talk of the town for quite a long time now and obviously for all the right reasons. Due to its high magnitude of health benefits, it enjoys the status of Heart-healthy by the Mayo Clinic. According to UNESCO, the Mediterranean diet has surpassed all the other diets in terms of health benefits and sustainability. In 2010, it recognized the Mediterranean diet as the "Cultural Heritage of The Mediterranean Countries" like Spain, Greece, Italy, and Morocco.

In 2020, the Mediterranean diet was voted the best diet of 2020 nutrition professionals. With all its popularity, many people have rushed to adopt the Mediterranean diet without fully understanding how it works and their efforts ended up in failure. This is because every diet faces a misconception. Saying farewell to your regular diet and switching completely to a different diet may lead to a whole new problem. The perceived help you get, in the form of articles, cookbooks, or dietitians, doesn't properly shed light on what the Mediterranean diet might mean, and obviously, the information is overwhelming. You are not sure of the right direction to follow. So here comes the very basic but burning question – WHAT EXACTLY IS THE MEDITERRANEAN DIET?!

Let's start with the word 'diet.' The word diet immediately makes you think of cutting down on food, counting calories and starving your stomach. That is the association we have been conditioned to because all the famous diets such as the Ketogenic diet and Atkins diet operate on low-carbs and high protein. These diets were created with the purpose of helping people lose weight. The latter diet helped people in their weight loss journey, but the weight was regained as soon as people switched to their normal eating habits. This is why the world needed a sustainable diet that could become a part of their lifestyle, and that's where the Mediterranean diet comes in.

The Mediterranean diet is not a diet at all but a lifestyle of the people living in Mediterranean countries. It is a culinary heritage of Mediterranean people that emphasizes the consumption of fresh fruits and seasonal vegetables. The Mediterranean diet is not about restricting food and does not focus on tracking calories. Instead, this lifestyle change aims to help you successfully eliminate unhealthy foods from your life while adding in more whole ones. It is also important to consider how these dietary changes affect habits and relationships with friends and family members. The Mediterranean diet emphasizes eating fresh seasonal foods grown locally. Whole grains, healthy fats, legumes, beans, fish, and dairy, make up a majority of the rest of the diet. Some Mediterranean regions incorporate a great deal more legumes and lentils, while others may enjoy more whole grains options. The similarity, however, is that all these regions enjoy plenty of plant-based foods and limit processed foods as well as added sugars and refined foods from their diets. Each region consumes nearly 2 to 3 times as many fruits and vegetables compared to those on the western diet. They also eat healthy fats like olive oil, nuts, and seeds regularly.

Important Features of the Mediterranean Diet

- A majority of the Mediterranean diet consists of fresh produce like organic fruits and vegetables.
- Whole grains like barley, millet, and whole-wheat add a unique flavor to your meal with their nutty texture. These nutritious grains are enjoyed as side dishes but could be incorporated into main courses too.
- Beans, lentils, and legumes make up a significant source of protein in the Mediterranean diet. These foods tend to make up for the limited consumption of red meats.
- Chicken, turkey, duck, and fish are good lean meat options that you can load up on your plate a few times per week. Lean meats (white meat) have lower calories and less saturated fats than red meat options. And that's why lean meats make the Mediterranean diet apt for weight reduction.
- Seafood such as scallops, shrimps, prawns, lobster e.t.c are incorporated into weekly meals at least twice a week.
- Another option for protein is red meat, but it should be the last option. This is because red meats contain saturated fat and cholesterol, which contribute to increased blood cholesterol levels and may cause heart ailments. So, have red meats only once a month and make sure they are grass-fed. A nice and delicious way to incorporate red meat in the Mediterranean diet is baking the meat with herbs and grill, not deep-frying.
- Drinking red wine in moderation is considered healthy on this diet and may help to lower the risk of heart disease. A glass or two per day has been shown to benefit your health overall.

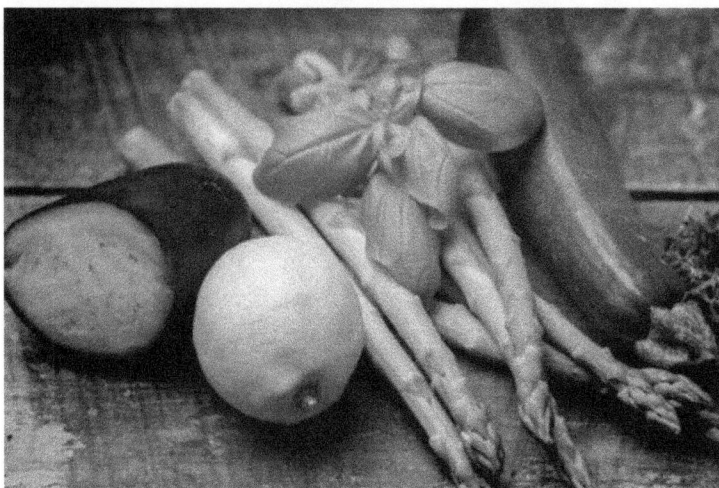

The History of the Mediterranean Diet

Many cultures have lived around the Mediterranean Sea, and their diet is important. One of their most important achievements has been the Mediterranean diet. It is hard to pinpoint where the Mediterranean originated since the eating habits that fall under this go far back into the Middle Ages.

People began farming in the areas surrounding the Mediterranean Sea, including countries like Lebanon, Israel, Palestine, Syria, and Jordan. They grew cereals and legumes. Later on, people from other countries came to live there, like Greeks and Romans. These people began to cultivate three basic food groups of the Mediterranean diet, such as olive trees for olive oil, wheat for bread, and grapevines, for the production of grapes and its main fermentation product, wine. The richer cast of Ancient Rome loved fresh fish and seafood with a special focus on oysters - either raw or fried in olive oil, while the middle or lower-middle class of Rome, including slaves, consumed foods that consisted of bread served with olive oil and olives, rarely eating any meat. (Altomare, 2013).

In the 8th Century, after Christ, Moors occupied Spain, they introduced new foods like rice and lemons to the area. These new foods gradually spread to the whole Mediterranean region. The occupation of the Moors ended in 1492, which is also when

Christopher Columbus came back from America with tomatoes and peppers. Since the 1960s, people have been interested in the eating habits of Mediterranean countries.

Scientific Research on the Mediterranean Diet

The first time people started investigating the Mediterranean diet was back in 1948 when a study was carried out on the constituents of the diet to prove its positive and negative impacts on overall health. This attempt was later rectified in 1952 by Ancel Keys, who sought to explore seven countries and their diet. The seven countries include the USA, Japan, Italy, Greece, Finland, the Netherlands, and Yugoslavia. The study spanned over three decades and evaluated data of 12,000 men aged 40 to 59. The results linked dietary intake with serum cholesterol levels and cardiovascular diseases, while low rates of cardiovascular diseases were linked to participants who had lower consumption of saturated fats. Another research conducted by the European Atomic Energy Commission, which took place from 1963 to 1965, sought to research the food consumption in 11 regions across six countries, nine regions in Northern Europe and two regions in Southern Europe. The only difference in their dietary patterns was in total fat intake where olive oil was its main source in the southern regions while butter was preferred in the northern regions. Margarine wasn't part of their diet and that's why the research found that the people in Northern and Southern Europe were also at less risk of suffering from chronic diseases. That is why, following this study, the potential effect of the Mediterranean diet, on reducing chronic diseases, was widely accepted. (Sahyoun, 2016)

After Ancel Keys, many people have conducted intensive research on the Mediterranean diet and its health benefits, including an increased lifespan, healthy weight, and improved brain function, fewer symptoms of rheumatoid arthritis, and eye health, lower risk of certain types of cancers, lower risk of heart disease, Alzheimer's, diabetes, and finally, lower blood pressure and LDL cholesterol levels. In fact, the Lyon Diet Trial proved that after three years of the continuous Mediterranean diet, the subjects showed a 50 percent lower risk of death and 50 to 70 percent reduced risk of myocardial infarction. Another research that gained worldwide attention was done by researchers in Spain who found that the Mediterranean diets, which included nuts, reduced the risk of cardiovascular diseases by 30 percent and decreased the risk of stroke by 49 percent. (Altomare, 2013)

From 2010 and onwards, many experts and doctors have recommended the Mediterranean diet for patients trying to lose weight or improve their overall wellbeing. Since then, it has been hailed as one of the best diets around. The amazing thing about the Mediterranean diet is that it doesn't credit one food or vegetable for the decreased health problems and weight loss but rather the whole plant-based diet with a special focus on local, regional, and locally available rich foods as a whole create a rich environment within the body and is responsible for all these reduced health problems. (Altomare, 2013)

As I have stated previously, the Mediterranean diet has been the focus of many research studies, and we already know about the multitude of health benefits it has. Aside from these, the Mediterranean diet is also used for weight loss. One research called "Mediterranean Diet and Weight Loss: Meta-Analysis of Randomized Controlled Trials" observed 1848 people on a Mediterranean diet and 1588 people on a controlled diet. The people who were following the Mediterranean diet showed a significant difference in weight and body mass index. The difference was observed mainly through energy restriction and increased physical activity. In no part of the study did any participant report gaining any weight, so through this study, we can conclude that the Mediterranean diet will be useful in losing weight, especially if it is accompanied by physical activity such as exercise and is longer than 6 months or is at least 6 months in duration. (Esposito, 2011)

Another research titled Systematic Review of the Mediterranean Diet for Long-Term Weight Loss supported the results of our previous research. It looked at the long-term benefits of the Mediterranean diet in obese and overweight participants. In the trials, the Mediterranean diet was compared to a low-fat diet, a low-carbohydrate diet, and the American diabetes association diet. The people in the Mediterranean diet group showed greater weight loss than the low-fat diet at 12 months. The Mediterranean diet also improved the cardiovascular risk factor levels, including blood pressure and lipid levels. (G. Mancini, 2016)

Over the last few decades, we have accumulated enough evidence that supports the fact that dietary habits have a large impact on the occurrence of diseases. The major scientific associations such as WHO, world health organization emphasize the role of diet in preventing non-communicable diseases. Many studies noticed that foods such as fruits and vegetables, fibers and whole grains with fish, and moderate alcohol consumption reduced the risk of major degenerative diseases and the food groups that are usually associated with that fall under the Mediterranean diet. Similarly, the Mediterranean diet

has been associated with a more favorable health outcome and a better quality of life. (Sofi, 2015)

The Mediterranean diet is created by a centuries-old tradition that is associated with excellent health and provides a sense of pleasure and wellbeing. It, in a sense, forms a vital part of the world's collective cultural heritage. The Mediterranean diet has several characteristics: an abundance of plant foods, olive oil as the principal fat, dairy products mostly yogurt and cheese, red meat, poultry, fish, and eggs in moderate amounts, moderate wine, and physical activity. For Mediterranean people, the diet is a way of living that needs to be revitalized in modern times, and people who want to follow such a diet are intrigued and attracted because of the strong palatability and the health benefits that are associated with the diet. The meals can be either recreated on their own or take into account different cultures and the feasibility of local ingredients. (Willet, 1995)

I want to believe that by now, you have successfully gathered "WHAT ACTUALLY A MEDITERRANEAN DIET IS." In the next chapter, you will find all the necessary information to satisfy your every possible "WHY THE MEDITERRANEAN DIET" question. I am sure that the research would be more than enough for you to easily incorporate the elements of the Mediterranean lifestyle diet into your life. You can even tailor the Mediterranean diet according to your native cuisine, and like me, you can also enjoy the best of both worlds!!!

Chapter 2

Mediterranean Lifestyle and Benefits

The major part of the Mediterranean lifestyle emphasizes the consumption of plant-based foods into your diet. The main components of the Mediterranean lifestyle include generous eating of fresh vegetables, fruits, legumes, whole grains, fish, and mindful consumption of dairy products, white and red meat. With these food options, the Mediterranean diet lifestyle ensures that your body gets all the required nutrients to keep it healthy and wealthy while boosting your immune system. Moreover, once the body's nutrient requirements have been achieved, you will naturally feel satiated, and therefore, will not feel the need to retreat to processed foods. This chapter will discuss the benefits of the Mediterranean lifestyle but before we go into that, it is important that you know the key food groups that make up the Mediterranean diet and make it apt to lead a healthy lifestyle.

Key Food Groups

➤ Vegetables

Fresh vegetables constitute a major part of the Mediterranean diet. To retain most of the nutrients and vitamins, vegetables are eaten uncooked or slightly cooked. Bitter green vegetables like spinach, kale, or broccoli are some of the nutritious veggies that are included in this diet. These vegetables are highly rich in Vitamin A, K, and C. Besides, vegetables are also loaded with high amounts of omega-3 fatty acids. These acids are proven to be extremely beneficial for improving digestion and mitigating the chances of constipation. The amazing thing about vegetables is the fact that they are always in the season. Thus, you are never going to run out of choices.

Most of the Mediterranean meals consist of the vegetables cooked in one or the other way, and on very rare occasions, meat is included; otherwise, it is all green on the plate. Perpetually on dinners, the vegetables are served as either grilled, sauteed, or roasted.

Sometimes, salads are eaten too, along with them served as side dishes. On this diet, picking vegetables is considered a serious matter. Habitants of Mediterranean regions grow their vegetable farms and then handpick the fresh and best ones. If you do not have a farm, then it is nothing to worry about. You can always go to the local vegetable shops as they receive fresh stock almost every day directly from the farms. The reason behind choosing organic and freshly grown vegetables is that they are highly rich in nutrients. Thus, it is evident that the Mediterranean diet is all about eating locally grown fresh vegetables. You might also go overboard and buy all the organic produce but never forget that you can always freeze the vegetables in plastic bags and use them when needed.

It is important to know that canned vegetables can never be the substitute for organically grown ones. Although they have all the characteristics to tempt you, like cheap prices and quick-cooking but very low in nutrients and contain extra salt/sugar added as preservatives. So, if you wholeheartedly want to adopt the Mediterranean lifestyle, you will have to part ways with canned foods. Still, you can always use canned veggies packed in water with little to no salt/sugar. In addition to the above facts, it is recommended that you bring diversity. Simply put, do not limit yourself to some specific vegetables; instead, eat whatever seasonal vegetables are available to you.

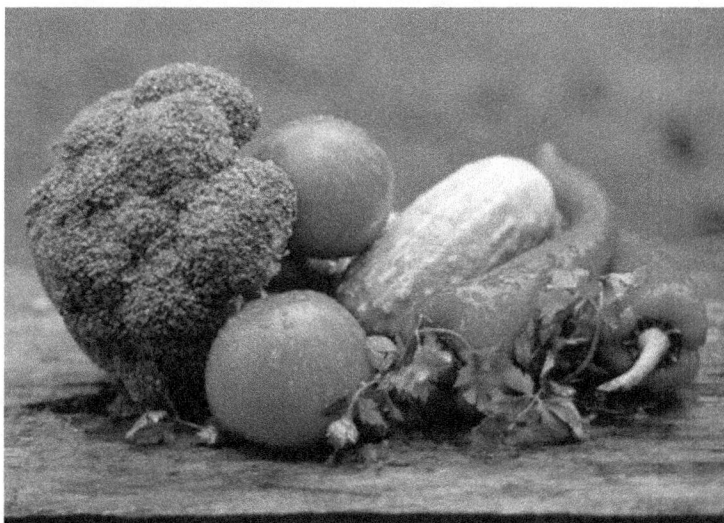

➢ Fruits

Regular fruit intake on the Mediterranean diet is a must. On this diet, fruits work as the replacement for desserts. They provide enough sugar rush that keeps you away from satisfying your sweet tooth with regular sugar-laden treats. Fruits are usually eaten for breakfast and sometimes as snacks, too, if hunger persists. Fruits can also be preserved or frozen to later use in ice cream and smoothies.

The Mediterranean diet also encourages the consumption of citrus fruits. Lemon juice is used as the most significant part of Mediterranean food. Its juice can be squished into your curry to give it a citric taste. There are no hard and fast rules to eat fruits that are purely grown in the Mediterranean region; the gist of the Mediterranean diet is to eat seasonal and fresh fruits that you can find locally in your region.

➢ Fats

The Mediterranean diet is primarily about using mono-saturated fats like olive oil. In simple terms, healthy fats. However, you should know that not all fats are similar and healthy. Some types of fats are very rich in bad cholesterol that can potentially destroy your heart health. While other types of fats are unsaturated and do not stick to your muscles, thereby reducing the chances of weight gain. Olive oil is one such example, which is the backbone of Mediterranean food, and that's why the majority of the Mediterranean recipes are cooked in olive oil. The reason is that olive oil helps with digestion and carries out maximum nutrient absorption, and helps you feel satiated.

The taste of olive oil varies from country to country. For example, olive oil in Mediterranean countries is flavorful and rich in taste. Whereas olive oil produced in America is slightly tasteless. But this must not excuse you from cooking your food in olive oil because of taste or no taste; it is healthy for you in many ways.

Besides, olive oil, another rich source of healthy fats on the Mediterranean diet, is driven from coconut, almonds, walnuts, and chia seeds. These nuts are rich in magnesium, vitamin E, and protein. Consuming enough of these nuts will ensure that you never end up in a hospital bed due to heart malfunction-related causes or diabetes.

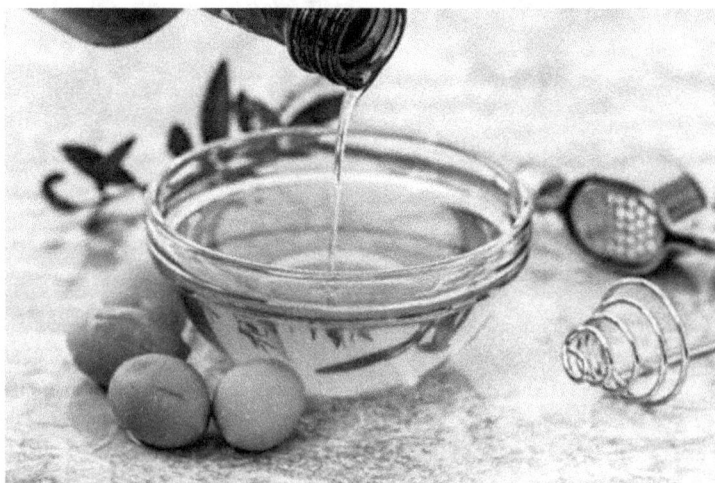

➢ Lentils

Legumes are the replacement for meat on the Mediterranean diet because they are a rich source of protein. It is seen that Mediterranean regions consume more lentils as compared to America; this is because many Mediterranean habitants observe fasts for quite a bit of time in the year, and during those days, they abstain from eating meat. This precisely explains the large consumption of lentils by Mediterranean people. Chickpeas, beans, and white beans are largely eaten on the Mediterranean diet, and these can easily be found in America. Contrary to people's belief, lentils are easy and quick to cook, given that you soak them for a while before cooking.

➢ Wholegrains

The fundamental components of the Mediterranean diet are whole grains. Whole grains include foods like bread, pasta, and rice. It is a cooking ritual in Mediterranean regions to always have a basket of bread placed during breakfast, lunch, and dinner for everyone to share from when they sit together at mealtimes. The bread usually consumed is made of sourdough, unlike white bread that is produced with the help of yeast. Furthermore,

barley and wheat are the most commonly used whole grains on the Mediterranean diet. The whole grains are served as side dishes cooked in vegetables and beans.

➢ Fish

As vegetables and fruits account for the major part of the Mediterranean diet, people often attribute this diet with no traces of seafood. But that is not true because the Mediterranean diet does allow the consumption of kinds of seafood like sardines, anchovies, but their servings are kept small and eaten only once or twice a week. Moreover, since fish has healthy oils, it has been given a separate category from red meats. Octopus and mussels are considered to be the delights of Mediterranean dinners. Their scrumptious taste makes the Mediterranean diet all more worth it.

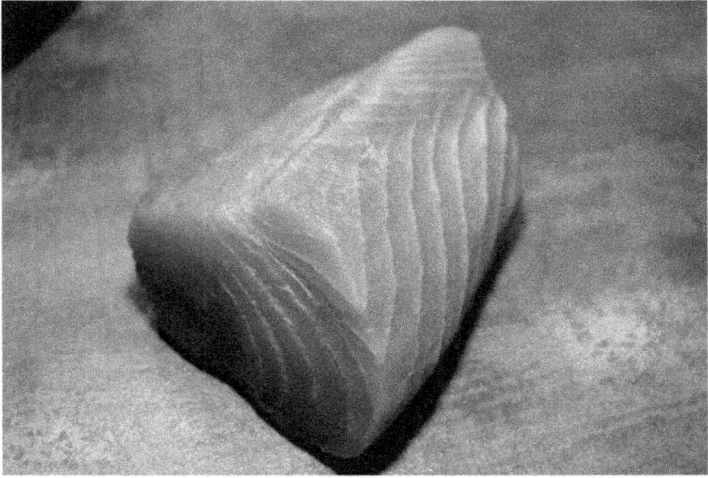

➤ Dairy

On a Mediterranean diet, consumption of dairy products is limited. Since milk and cheese tend to be high in cholesterol, their usage has been restricted to once or twice a week. By now, we know that the Mediterranean diet is all about keeping one healthy and fit, so how can it possibly allow the consumption of such fats that can potentially form fat clots in heart arteries causing a heart attack or leading to obesity. So instead, preference is given low-fat dairy items or made from plants such as almond and coconut milk, coconut yogurt, etc.

➤ Red Meat

Red meat is only eaten on special occasions when on the Mediterranean diet. It is served as a side dish instead of the main course. The servings are kept small. Its replacement includes fish, poultry, and beans. The meat of grass-fed animals can also be a viable replacement for red meat primarily because the earlier animals are healthier and eat clean. The best recommendation by the dietician is that when you want to choose meat, choose one that is 90 percent lean with 10 percent fat.

You will get more details about making your plate for the Mediterranean diet as per serving in the section "The Mediterranean Diet Food List" of chapter 3.

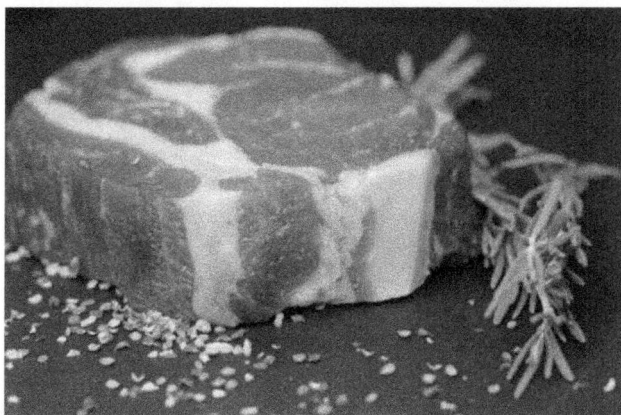

Mealtimes are Get-Together Times

Mediterranean meals are seen as a way to relax and reconnect. They transform mealtimes into an experience, encouraging family members to gather at the table for conversation instead of staying on their phones or watching T.V. in another room. In the western world, many are used to rushing through meals as fast as possible. We often approach this experience with an obligation rather than a time for reflection and connection. It is common in American homes for family members to be glued to their phones scrolling social media during dinner times. This lack of engagement leads to increased stress levels, leading one to depression or other mental health issues over long periods. An alternative solution would be putting down your devices at mealtime instead and focusing on those around you, enjoying them more fully - it will reduce stress and increase moods overall. Social eating or the act of sharing a meal with another person can reduce stress and the risk of overeating. Eating together as a family is also an opportunity to connect and support your children while also teaching them how to eat healthily.

Even though cooking is usually a solitary event, it has also been known to be social. When multiple people get together in the kitchen, they can connect and share their days' events. It is not uncommon for those invited over dinner to come early so that everyone can help cook and stay connected throughout the night.

Exercise is the Key

The Mediterranean region is an area where physical activity plays a major role in the health of its citizens. Many people there choose to walk rather than drive or take public transit all around their cities and towns. And this leads them closer with neighbors and friends. Not only that, but these regular walks play a large part in exceptional wellbeing for those who live here. Most individuals who follow the Mediterranean diet also get two hours of cardio or aerobic exercise per week. It can be split up throughout the week and done in 10-minute intervals by engaging in daily chores such as mowing your lawn, cleaning the house, vacuuming carpets, etc. You can also divide it by exercising at least two hours per week by running around with your kids for fun or even dancing.

Some exercises to consider:

- Jogging
- Swimming
- Yoga
- Running
- Walking
- Strength training
- Resistance training
- Cycling

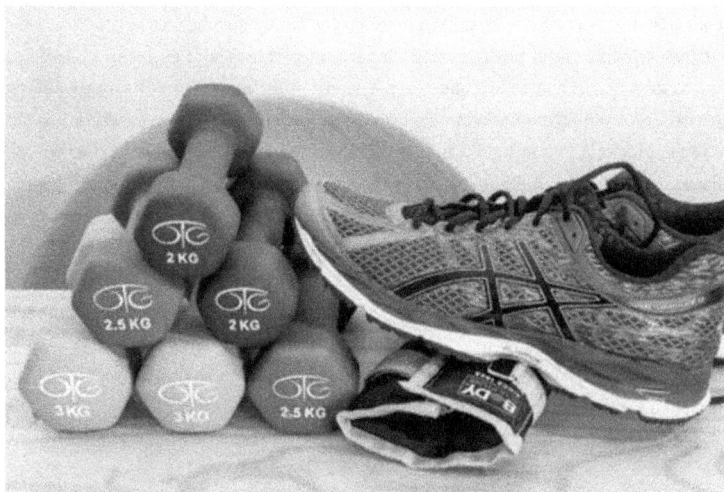

Health Benefits of the Mediterranean Diet

Let's talk about the impact of the Mediterranean lifestyle on our health. As you are aware now, the Mediterranean diet focuses on eating a variety of fruits, vegetables, nuts, healthy fats, and proteins. This healthy lifestyle has been proven to increase life expectancy by up to 10 years! Along with the benefits for your health, adopting this diet can also provide increased mental clarity because it is high in Omega-3s, which support brain function. So, if you are looking for improved mood or decreased anxiety levels, then look no further than changing how you eat. Seriously, what could be better?

The significant health benefits of the Mediterranean diet can be found below:

➤   *Strengthens Heart Health*

A large clinical trial in Spain of 7,000 people with pre-diabetes or high risk for cardiovascular disease showed that those who ate a calorie-unrestricted Mediterranean diet rich in olive oil and nuts had at least a 30 percent lower chance of heart attack. So undoubtedly, the Mediterranean diet is a wholesome, healthy way to reduce the risk of cardiovascular disease.

➤   *Minimize Women's Risk for Stroke*

A September 2018 study published in the Stroke Journal found that following a Mediterranean diet could lower the risk of stroke, especially for women at high risk. Researchers examined data on 23,232 men and women ages 40 to 77 from the United Kingdom, with most being white. The results showed a significant reduction in strokes only for female participants, not so much among males. Females experienced an average 20 percent decrease when they followed this specific diet regimen closely.

➤   *Good For Cognitive and Prevention of Brain Damage*

To provide the brain with all of its nutritional needs, people must have a rich blood supply. However, those who are experiencing vascular issues can experience significant cognitive decline as well. A July 2016 review published in the journal Frontiers in Nutrition examined studies that looked at cognitive function and concluded: "*there is encouraging evidence that a higher adherence to the Mediterranean diet improves cognition, slows cognitive decline or reduces conversion from Alzheimer's disease."*

> ➤ *Keeps Cancer at Bay*

The Mediterranean diet plan is considered very effective in mitigating the chances of developing certain types of cancers, such as breast cancer. New research has shown that the Mediterranean diet can help reduce your risk of breast cancer and colorectal cancers and prevent death from these types of cancer.

The Mediterranean diet is linked to lower rates of depression, according to a study published in September 2018. Analysis from four longitudinal studies revealed that the reduction was 33 percent.

> ➤ *Weight Loss on the Mediterranean Diet*

The Mediterranean diet, by far, provides an authentic and sure way to shed extra pounds naturally and easily. Unlike other diets like keto diets that follow the principle of low carbohydrates and more protein, the Mediterranean diet strikes a balance between all the basic nutrients required by the human body.

It does not deprive you of food like other diets; instead, it provides you with healthy food rich in antioxidants that stimulate fast metabolism, thereby quick digestion and no fat storage. In addition to that, the Mediterranean diet is clean eating where you are cutting off the sources of bad cholesterol that leads to obesity. Also, it removes fast foods from your life which are the big cause of obesity in people. The latter ensures lower calorie intake and quick satiation. Since the Mediterranean diet is rich in healthful foods and provides a high quantity of fiber and good fats, both of these lead to weight loss.

With all the information for understanding the prominent features of the Mediterranean lifestyle along with food groups and potential health advantages, it's time to dive a little deeper to comprehend your adaptation to it. The efforts you need to make for **TRANSITIONING TO THE MEDITERRANEAN DIET** are convenient and a lot easier than you can imagine!

Chapter 3

Planning your Mediterranean Diet

L ike I discussed with you at the beginning of chapter 1, many people dive right into this new way of eating without planning or understanding the ins and outs of what they should be doing to achieve their goals. That is precisely what this chapter is about – planning your Mediterranean diet plate, convenient steps to get started with the diet, a detailed food list, and tricks for ensuring your success in adapting to the Mediterranean diet.

So, the transition to the diet can get a lot easier, and for this, it is necessary to gather all the information about the ingredients and their cooking techniques to make this transition easy and smooth. In addition, you should know what foods to eat, what foods to avoid and what foods to not eat at all. Even though there are no supplements or special foods to purchase, some key ingredients are a must-have on this diet, which you will be required to buy and stock up on. Moreover, you will also have to locate organic farms that could supply fresh stock of seasonal fruits and vegetables.

Transitioning to the Mediterranean diet is mostly about making yourself ready for a new way of eating. It also means adapting to the Mediterranean lifestyle and changing your relationship with food. For this journey to be merry, you will have to unlearn everything about your unhealthy eating habits and change how you look at food. It suffices to say that transitioning to the Mediterranean diet demands a change of mindset and modifying your life so that the Mediterranean diet becomes your natural eating pattern. You can take as much time as you want to prepare yourself beforehand.

Planning Your Mediterranean Diet

Unlike other fancy diets, you do not have to run stores to stores to get the right ingredients to prepare a Mediterranean dish. Ingredients of the Mediterranean diet are available almost everywhere. You are also not required to buy advanced electrical appliances to cook your food into. The only thing you have to do is find the right ingredients and get started. You need to take care of just a few things, and you will be

successful on this diet. The following are some of the ways you can start mentally preparing yourself for transitioning to the Mediterranean diet.

➤   *Make Healthy Eating Effortless*

Before completely diving into the Mediterranean eating patterns, it is advisable to cut off all ties with processed, unhealthy foods. This will serve as a warm-up for you. If this goes smoothly, then you will not have much problem adjusting to the said diet. Start by completely boycotting fast foods. Then slowly start cutting on other processed food like chips, canned and frozen foods.

You can also snub on processed drinks like sodas, juices, and coffee and replace them with milk, butter, sugar. As far as frozen meat is concerned, you can replace it with a limited portion of red meat.

It may seem overwhelming to abruptly cut down these foods because your body has been using them as a source of energy for a long time. This is why it needs to be done slowly and gradually. After some time of following this regime, you will notice positive changes in your body.

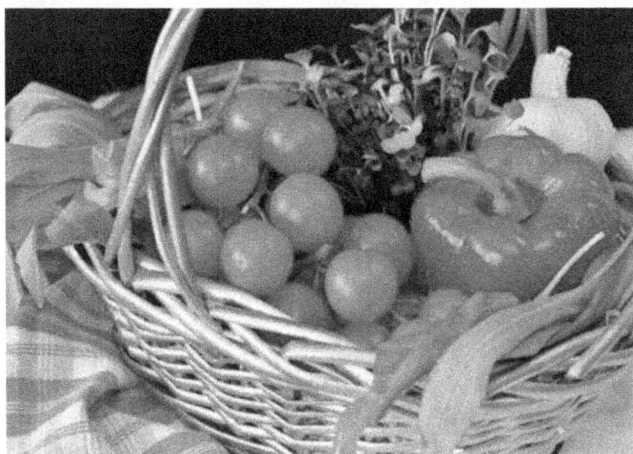

➤   *Think About the Scrumptious Mediterranean Food*

Think of Mediterranean food as like going on a vacation. When you plan for a trip, you do your homework beforehand, for example, searching for hotels, places to visit, and things to try. It builds a certain excitement and gives you a reason to look forward to. Just like that, consider practicing the Mediterranean diet as an adventure and a quest for attaining maximum health benefits. Therefore, you should educate yourself about everything related to the Mediterranean diet, for example, foods and drinks to have and avoid. Plus, cooking Mediterranean dishes will take this adventure to another level; see chapter 5 and onwards to try your cooking skills. In this manner, you will train yourself enough to ensure a successful and smooth transition.

➤   *Shop For the Ingredients*

The best part about the Mediterranean diet is that the ingredients used in it are readily available everywhere, be it supermarkets, organic farms, or even your backyard garden. Chapter 2 discussed the importance of picking your own produce, and for this, you need to make this activity a joyful quest.

All you need to do is put your coat on and be on your way to get fresh vegetables and fruits. Of course, you will have to check out the freshness and get a quote for prices too. In this manner, you will be better equipped to shop for your required ingredients. Still, the primary goal is to locate as many sources of fresh fruits, vegetables, and meat regardless of the time taken in the process. The most recommended way to source your food on the Mediterranean diet is to source it from organic farms. These farms produce fresh and healthy seasonal food. This food is not only rich in nutrition, but it tastes good as well. Also, try to befriend the vendors, so you can remain updated about the upcoming stock. You can also talk to farmers and inquire about the timings of harvests of different vegetables used on the Mediterranean diet. Befriending farmers, talking to them, and taking an interest in what they do is an amazing way to encourage healthy social interaction. The latter is part of Mediterranean culture. Besides friendship, you can get amazing discounts and updated information on the upcoming harvests too. And as you get used to shopping, the experience will be just like a trip to the park.

You can also retreat to supermarkets and grocery stores if you cannot access local farms. As long as you abide by the basic notions of the Mediterranean diet, you are on the right track. While shopping for Mediterranean ingredients, try to stay in the vicinity of the market. It implies that you should try to buy all of your ingredients from the fresh produce section, including seafood, dairy, and meat. Fill your cart with as many organic fruits and vegetables as you can because you can never have enough healthy food. These vegetables are going to be a rich source of antioxidants for you. Moreover, try to opt for in-season fruits rather than out-season. The reason is that out-season fruits usually have lost their nutritional value.

Befriend the sea monger at the seafood shop. Do this for two reasons. Firstly, you get to fill your cart with fresh fish; and secondly, he will be able to help you pick the fresh fish and even, could share scrumptious Mediterranean cooking recipes with you—all the good reasons to be friends with them. Try to choose cold water fishes as they are rich in omega-3. For example, you can go for sardines, salmon, mackerel, and cod.

In addition to that, avoid shopping for food from center aisles in the supermarkets, as these sells processed and artificial preserved canned foods, which is a big no on the Mediterranean diet. What you can only get from these aisles are oils and whole grains like pasta, bread, and walnuts. Just to be sure, keep your grocery list in hand so you don't get tempted by forbidden foods on this diet.

Steps to Get Started with the Mediterranean Diet

The primary proposition of the Mediterranean diet is to replicate the eating pattern of the Mediterranean regions. The U.S. Department of Agriculture's (USDA) My plate provides a comprehensive guideline in the "Dietary Guidelines for Americans 2020-2025" about eating healthy foods on the Mediterranean diet. You can go through the details according to your age group; however, if you still feel confused about food choices, then remember one simple rule and apply it to every meal. Make half your plate fruits and vegetables, one-quarter of your plate whole grains, one-quarter of your plate healthy protein, some dairy, and lots of water.

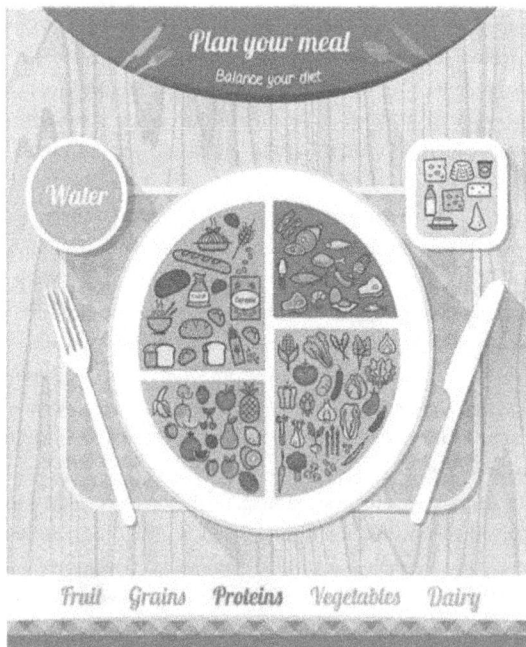

The Mediterranean lifestyle is an easy way to get back on track with your healthy eating habits. It has been found that people who live in this region have lower obesity, heart disease, and diabetes rates than the average person. Therefore, the Mediterranean diet is a great choice for anyone looking to get healthier, lower cholesterol levels, and lose weight. Now that you have been introduced to the wonders of a Mediterranean diet, it is time to show you how easy and delicious transitioning into this lifestyle can be. I will walk you through a five-step guide for making the switch from your old ways with healthy eating habits so come along on an exciting journey toward better health.

I have mentioned five steps for your ease in transitioning to the Mediterranean diet.

Step 1: When You Cook, Use Olive Oil

You must replace other fats with olive oil if you want the benefits of the Mediterranean diet. Olive oil is central to this type of diet, and many people think it has good fats. But, if you do not replace other types of fat with olive oil, then you will not get those benefits.

Step 2: Eat Vegetables as the Main Dish

One of the main features that set the Mediterranean Diet apart from most other diets is its high consumption of vegetables. Greeks consume almost a pound per day, and this can be seen in their cooking techniques, such as sautéed green beans with olive oil or tomato sauce.

Step 3: Learn to Cook Some Simple Mediterranean Meals

The Mediterranean diet is a refreshing change from the Western standard. It consists of real food that can make your life happier and healthier, like omelets with fresh vegetables or grilled fish topped with tomatoes. You might not have to cook from scratch every day, but learning 2-3 basic dishes will help you in the long run.

Step 4: Try Going Vegan for One Day A Week

It may have been that the Greeks' diet was so healthy because they abstained from animal products for roughly half of their year. This would make sense as not only a religious practice but also potentially an important factor in why this population had much better health than others at the time due to less consumption of animal-based foods and more plant-based foods.

Step 5: Do Not Add Meat to Everything

Many people see vegetables on the recommendation list, but what does meat add to a diet? Studies show that reducing your intake of red and white meats will have better health benefits. Try these guidelines: one serving of lean beef once per week and three servings of chicken weekly, one every two days, with fish as an alternative for those who do not like white or red meat.

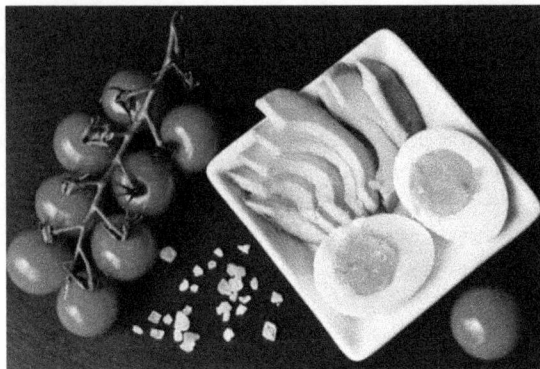

The Mediterranean Diet Food List

The Mediterranean diet is often considered a way to promote good health and longevity. The beauty of this dietary regimen lies in its never-ending food options, which, combined with the diversity of all regions, makes it rich. We need to take care of some basics when following or creating any type of Mediterranean style eating habits, such as what foods you should eat, which items to avoid, which beverages to drink, etc.

Vegetables
What to Eat liberally:

- All vegetables that are non-starchy such as dark greens, artichokes, eggplant, bell peppers, zucchini, etc.
- Brightly colored veggies such as kale, spinach, tomatoes, eggplant, squash, and okra.
- Moderately starchy vegetables such as root vegetables like carrots, beets, and sweet potatoes.
- Frozen or canned vegetables with no added sugar or salt.

What to Eat Rarely or Never:

- Vegetables that are very starchy such as white potatoes and corn.

Instructions for Servings:
At least 5 or more servings of fresh vegetables per day, such as

- make 2 servings of salad
- 1 medium vegetable
- ½ cup of canned vegetables
- 1 cup of leafy greens

Fruits

What to Eat liberally:

- All fruits that are high in fiber and low in sugar are allowed, such as berries, cherries, apricots, peaches, dates, oranges, pears, figs, melons, peaches, etc.
- Frozen or canned fruits with no added sugar or salt.
- Dried fruits with no added sugar.

What to Eat Rarely or Never:

- There is no fruit that is off-limit on the Mediterranean diet as long as it is fresh.

Instructions for Servings:

At least 3 or more servings of fresh fruit per day, such as

- have 1 medium fruit
- ½ cup of canned fruit
- ¼ cup dried fruit

Nuts and Seeds

What to Eat liberally:

Eat nuts and seeds but in moderation

What to Eat Occasionally:

- Almonds, pistachios, and cashews
- Walnuts and Hazelnut
- All unsweetened nuts

What to Eat Rarely or Never:

- Sugar-coated nuts
- Sweetened nut butter
- Sweetened trail mixes

Instructions for Servings:

- 1 serving of ¼ cup unsalted seeds or nuts per week

Whole Grains

What to Eat liberally:

- All grains that have whole or whole-grain in their name, including whole-grain wheat, whole-grain rice, etc.
- Products with whole grains as their first grain ingredients, such as whole-grain bread and whole-grain cereal
- Other grains and products include couscous, oats, barley, quinoa, bulgur, brown rice, wild rice, spelt, millet, farro, and buckwheat.

What to Eat Occasionally:

- Couscous
- Whole-wheat pasta
- Whole-grain crackers
- Polenta
- All-bran cereals

What to Eat Rarely or Never:

- Pancake mix
- Frozen waffles
- Sugar-sweetened cereals
- Crackers
- High fat snack foods like French fries, chips, buttered popcorn, cheese puffs, etc.

Instructions for Servings:

5 servings per day such as

- have ½ cup cooked grains in the form of rice or pasta
- 1 slice of wholegrain bread
- 30 grams of crackers or cold cereal
- ¾ cup hot cereal
- ½ of whole-grain roti, tortilla, or pita bread

Lentils, Beans, and Peas

What to Eat liberally:

- Red beans, kidney beans, and other beans, all lentils and pulses

Instructions for Servings:

At least 3 or more servings per week

- Make ¾ cup of cooked lentils, beans, and peas

Poultry and Red Meat

What to Eat liberally:

- Chicken, turkey, duck, game hens, eggs, and egg whites
- Plant-based alternatives of poultry such as tofu, tempeh, and seitan

What to Eat Occasionally:

- Red meat, grass-fed: beef, pork, lamb, or goat (baked, grilled)
- Bacon, grass-fed
- Processed meat products such as chicken nuggets (baked)

What to Eat Rarely or Never:

- Processed meat like ham, bacon, sausages, deli meats
- Meat cuts that are high in salt and saturated fats

Instructions for Servings:

- 2 to 5 servings of poultry per week
- 3 to 5 servings of red meat per month
- Prefer poultry to red meat

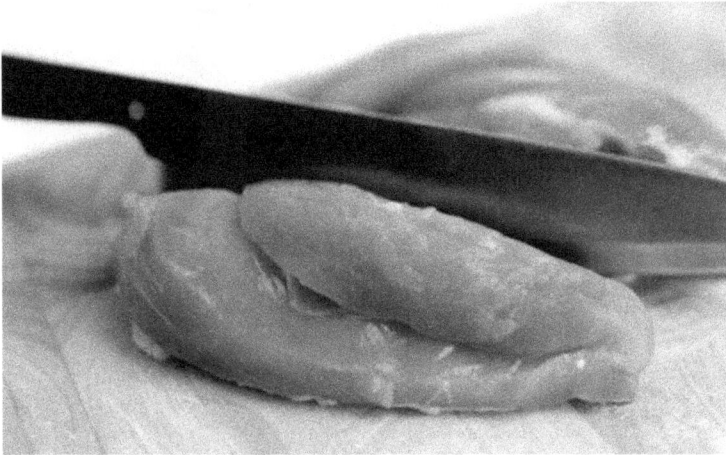

Fish and Seafood

What to Eat liberally:

- Fish that are high in omega-3 such as salmon, sardines, herring, mackerel, or trout
- Fresh, Frozen, or canned fish or seafood without added sugar or salt

Instructions for Servings:

At least 1 or 3 servings per week

- Have 100 grams (3.5 ounces) of fish

Dairy and Alternatives

What to Eat liberally:

- Milk, kefir, and yogurt that are low-fat and with little or no added sugar
- Plant-based milk and yogurt such as almond milk, coconut milk, hazelnut milk, coconut yogurt
- Cheese with less than 20 percent milk fat

What to Eat Occasionally:

- Milk
- Plain Greek yogurt
- Cottage cheese and ricotta cheese
- Brie cheese, goat cheese, feta cheese, etc.

What to Eat Rarely or Never:

- High-fat milk, butter, and cream
- Sweetened yogurt
- Ice cream
- All processed cheese

Instructions for Servings:
1 to 3 servings per day, such as

- Have 1 cup milk (1% or skim)
- ¾ cup kefir or low-fat yogurt
- 50 grams (1.5 ounces) cheese (less than 20 percent milkfat)

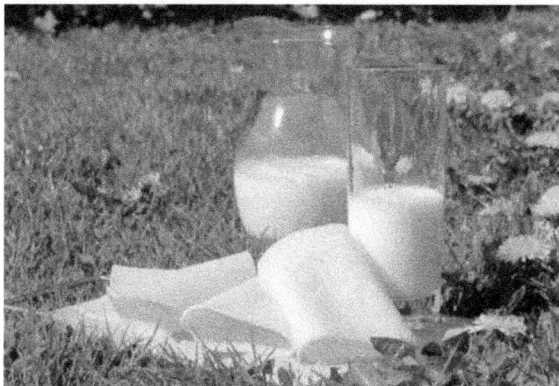

Oil and Fats

What to Eat liberally:

- Avocado and Olives
- Virgin or extra-virgin oil
- Plant-based oil such as coconut oil and avocado oil
- Seeds and nut butter

What to Eat Occasionally:

- Canola oil and soybean oil

What to Eat Rarely or Never:

- Butter
- Trans-fat
- Margarine

Instructions for Servings:

- At least 4 tablespoons or more oil per day at the table or in cooking
- 7 large or 10 small olives per week
- ½ of a medium avocado per week
- 2 tablespoons of seeds and nut butter per week

Sweeteners

What to Eat liberally:

- Consume sweeteners in moderation

What to Eat Occasionally:

- Coconut sugar
- Honey, agave syrup

What to Eat Rarely or Never:

- White sugar

Instructions for Servings:

- 1 to 3 teaspoons per day

Sauces and Condiments
What to Eat liberally:

- Tomato sauce without any sugar
- Pesto sauce, fresh
- Balsamic and apple cider vinegar

What to Eat Occasionally:

- Tzatziki sauce
- Tahini dip
- Aioli

What to Eat Rarely or Never:

- Sweetened sauces such as barbecue sauces
- Teriyaki sauce
- Ketchup

Instructions for Servings:

- 3 to 5 tablespoons per day

Beverages
What to Eat liberally:

- Water
- Green tea and low-fat tea with less sugar
- Coffee with less sugar, decaf coffee

What to Eat Occasionally:

- Red wine
- Other Alcohol

What to Eat Rarely or Never:

- Bottled fruit juices or drinks sweetened with sugar
- Iced tea
- Sweetened coffee
- Soda

Instructions for Servings:

- Women: no more than 2 drinks per day
- Men: no more than 3 drinks per day

1 drink is 5 ounces (142 ml) of drink/wine

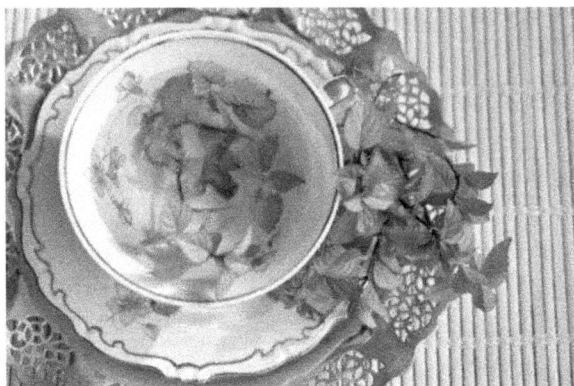

Tips For Success on The Mediterranean Diet

➤   *Eat-In A Way That Is Mindful and Moderate*

The Mediterranean Diet is different from other eating plans because it allows you to have some foods high in fat while still being healthy. Eating this way can also make your brain healthier and help reduce risk factors for heart disease. It is not about starving yourself or cutting out entire food groups; instead, eat moderately without going overboard on certain foods, especially sweets.

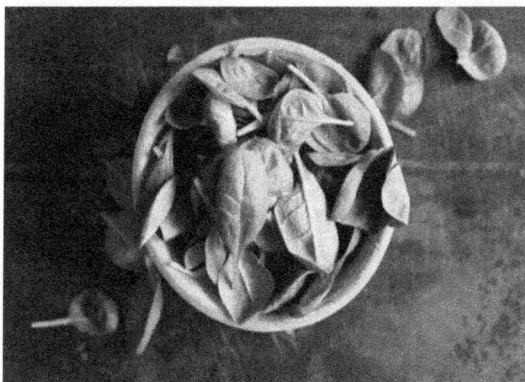

➤ *Find "Gateway" Fruits and Vegetables*

If you do not usually eat a lot of fresh produce, it might be hard to just start eating an apple or broccoli. But there are some vegetables that most people like: gateway vegetables or fruits. You just need to find the one that works for you and start eating that every day. And then, you can gradually go on to other healthy Mediterranean foods like tomatoes, cucumbers, green peppers, and carrots. It might take a year or more before the change happens, but it is worth it because you will feel better. Take it from my experience of losing weight with the Mediterranean diet; this book will help you lose weight in 30 days; however, I would suggest adopting the Mediterranean lifestyle for a year for effective results.

➤ *Include Signature Ingredients*

Tasty food is the best way to make your diet enjoyable. The Mediterranean diet is popular because it has ingredients that everyone likes. You can find recipes from around the Mediterranean that use the same signature ingredients, such as olive oil, whole grains, and vegetables. For protein, use fish, chicken, or a limited amount of red meat. You can create your own collection of Mediterranean dishes. Check out chapter 5 and onwards for inspiration.

➤ *Incorporate Weight Loss Components*

The Mediterranean diet is not only for weight loss as it is good for keeping the body fit, and healthy but it still plays a major role in weight loss. For effective weight loss, you need to restrict your portions and calories so you can lose some weight. Simple kitchen tools will help with this, like measuring spoons and a food scale. In addition, free apps and websites like myfitnesspal and cronometer will help you figure out how many of the right foods you should eat in a day. It might even make it easier for you to tailor healthy Mediterranean-style meals. A good thumb rule is to plan your meals of 1200 calories or less in total.

> *Treat Meals like a Social Event*

As discussed before, as an important element of the Mediterranean lifestyle, it is common to consider meal times as social events, where all friends and family members get to sit, talk and share laughs. A good human company is all that we need at the end of the day. By adopting a Mediterranean diet, we are going to increase our chances of social freedom and happiness. And, since everyone on the table will be eating the same diet food, this can motivate sticking to the Mediterranean diet for the long run as everyone will understand each other's struggle to live a hearty life. Moreover, you can learn by sharing your experiences with the respective health goals. Even your friend circle could serve as an accountable group to keep a check on each other's diet regime.

> *Eat with Concentration*

We often grab a bite on the go in our fast-paced lives because otherwise, we don't have time. Either we remain immersed in the work or occupied with other professional commitments. With such a lifestyle, we barely get a chance to truly enjoy our meal. But in the Mediterranean regions, people gather on dining tables and keep their phones aside; they truly focus on their food while interacting with other fellows.

> *Exercise is a Must*

For longer positive impacts on your mental and physical health, you need to continue your physical activity. Although any activity involving moving your body is welcome, you can always go for a walk with a friend or family. The reason is that it has been linked with improved heart health, weight loss, and better mental health.

➤   *Resist Temptation*

It is fairly common to stray away when you are on a diet. For example, you may feel a sudden craving for fried foods like French fries. It is at that point you should remember why you began this journey towards a healthy lifestyle. And, there is always a healthy alternative for your craving, for example, roasted sweet potato fries. Also, always keep healthy snacks within your reach. Munching these nutritious snacks will not only help you resist temptation but also keep you motivated and consistent.

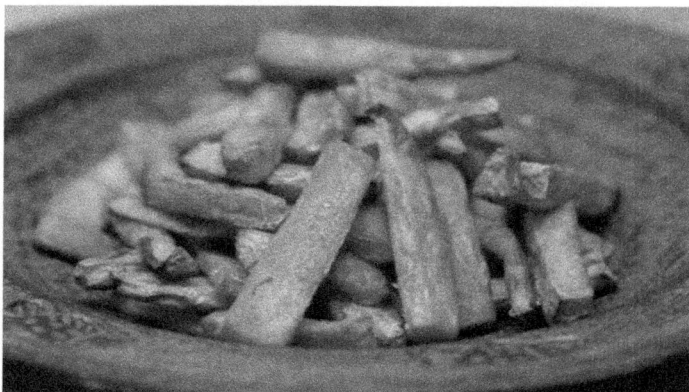

➤   *Do not Overwhelm Yourself*

When we start something new, our energy levels are always at a peak, but our motivation starts to wear down with time. This is normal because it is okay to fail first when you

abandon your decade-old unhealthy eating habits. But you should remind yourself that your older self will thank you for trying so hard to keep your body healthy.

Chapter 4

What to look out for in your Mediterranean Diet

Eating Out on The Mediterranean Diet

The Mediterranean diet is an easy-breezy diet, unlike other diets that limit your food intake and make you starve. This diet offers versatile food options from vegetables to meat. The only restriction it exerts is on the quantity of consumption and style of cooking the food. Our mouths get filled with water at the sight of scrumptious foods, especially if it is at a restaurant, but stopping yourself from eating it just because your diet regime does not permit it, is heartbreaking. No matter the circumstances, sometimes all we want is to eat what our heart desires. The good thing about the Mediterranean diet is the fact that it does not deprive you of any food, as long as it is fresh, organic, and unprocessed.

So, eating out on the Mediterranean diet is easier than you think. The healthier food groups' especially vegetarian food, provide one with enough options to choose from. Ever since the popularity of the Mediterranean diet, many restaurants have updated and modified their menus according to the standards of a Mediterranean diet. Is it not amazing? To be able to eat your favorite food at your favorite eatery without minding calories sure sounds like a dream come true.

Some of the best restaurants for people on the Mediterranean diet could be offering fresh organic farm food and seafood. As the Mediterranean diet is based on the eating habits of Mediterranean countries, so any restaurant serving Italian, Spanish, Greek, or Southern French foods can also compensate for restaurant food cravings. Many vegetarian restaurants serve the best Mediterranean food for you to try. If you happen to notice, a lot of vegetarian restaurants have food options closer to Mediterranean food groups. If you want to satisfy your food cravings while maintaining your diet regime, you must evaluate the frequency of the times you eat out. The reason is that such self-evaluation will assist you in finding a middle ground and help you decide the number of dinners you can afford in a week.

Here are some guidelines you can incorporate in your life and strictly follow when dining out on the Mediterranean diet.

Make Food Choices Based on Overall Diet

You need to ask yourself a simple question to base your food choices surrounding the Mediterranean diet; ask yourself how big part of your diet involves eating out? For example, if you eat once or twice a month, you have nothing to worry about. But if you happen to eat out twice or thrice in a week, then you definitely need to cut it short. Otherwise, there is no point in following the Mediterranean diet.

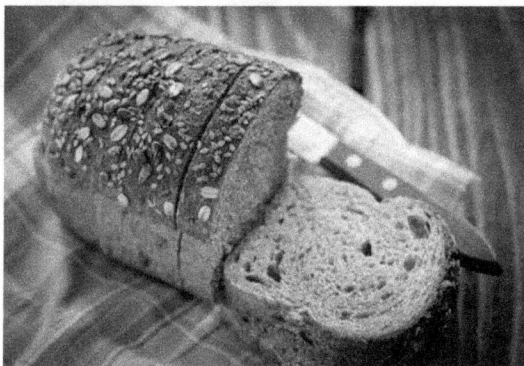

Eat Bread but Mindfully

Although bread is an integral food on a Mediterranean diet, you need to hold your taste buds until the main course is served. By munching on the bread only, you gain substantial calories, minimize your appetite, and deprive yourself of the main meal. This is why the Mediterranean diet preaches minimalism, suggesting that we eat everything healthy but in a limited amount.

Keep A Vegetarian Entrée as A Backup

It is part of human nature to lose interest and feel the urge to give up on a diet regime. Therefore, following and sticking to a diet requires a strong commitment. Still, along the way, you must expect the meltdowns and urges to terminate the Mediterranean regime. It is at this point; vegetarian entrée can save you from succumbing to processed foods. Vegetarian entrées serve plant-based foods containing all the essential nutrients of Mediterranean food, therefore preventing you from giving up the diet and simultaneously satisfying your taste buds.

Look For Boiled and Baked Food on The Menu

You need to securitize the menu thoroughly and look for food that's either boiled or baked. Make sure that the food is sautéed in olive oil instead of butter. Besides that, avoid deep-fried food.

Satisfy Your Craving for Alcoholic Drinks with Wine

Wine is the only alcoholic drink allowed on the Mediterranean diet, with 4-ounce or less per day for women and 8-ounce or less for men.

Always Leave Half Course on The Plate

It may sound unethical and brutal given you are a foodie, but always try to eat half of the food on the plate and then pause for a while. After a few moments, you won't feel as hungry as you were before. This is because it is common for people to go overboard on their cheat meals and throw everything in their stomach, although the hunger could be fulfilled with much less food. Therefore, it is better to eat until half of your stomach is filled, and then, you can get the remaining food parceled and eat the leftovers the next day.

Order Fish Salads

When eating out, try to include fish salad as a side dish beside the main course. Skip the creamy toppings and retreat to the olive oil and vinegar.

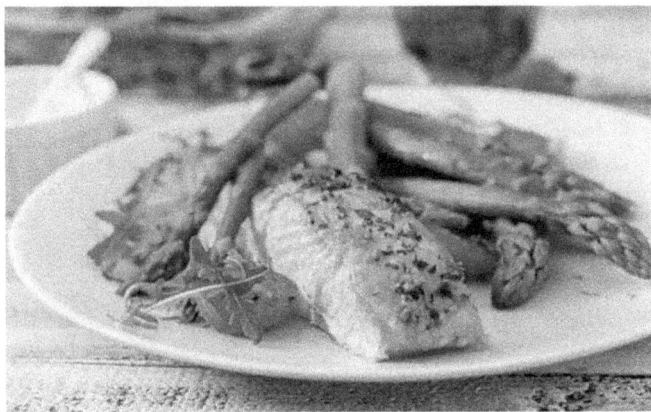

Let The Oil Slide

Most of the time, when we eat out, we do not know what cooking oil is used in the food. To address the latter problem, you can simply try asking the staff if the food is cooked in olive oil or not. If not, then you can either opt for baked dishes or the ones cooked in minimum oil.

Sweet Treats

As far as the desert is concerned, you can skip the scrumptious brownies and pastries and trade them with a plate of fruit salad, cheese, or other low-fat and Mediterranean diet-friendly desserts. The other options for desserts include a slice of chocolate cake or crème Brule.

As discussed in previous chapters, meal times in the Mediterranean diet are considered social events, where everyone gathers at one table and eats together while talking and laughing with one another. This makes dining out at restaurants a natural component of the Mediterranean diet; hence there is no need to stress where and what to eat. You are only required to keep one thing in mind, eat whatever you like but in a controlled amount. Besides that, most of the restaurants make food that is Mediterranean diet-friendly, so you do not have to worry at all.

Now, let's get on to the euphoric experience of Mediterranean-style cooking. In the next section, you will have a meal plan for 30 days. To see the result of the efforts you will put in for weight loss or keep it off, it is important to adopt and follow the Mediterranean diet for a minimum of 30 days. And that's why I have designed meals that give a maximum of 1200 total calories per day as this promotes weight loss. You will find healthy recipes for filling breakfasts, comforting lunches, quick-to-make snacks, hearty dinners, and decadent desserts. And last but not least, some Mediterranean sauces, salad dressings, and dips to maximize the flavors and make your meals extra-tasty!

Feel free to adjust the serving of recipes and experiment with food choices according to your taste and needs.

30 Days Meal Plan

Week 1

Day 1

Breakfast – Greek-Style Frittata (224 calories)

Lunch – Tuna Patties (216 calories)

Snack – Pineapple and Green Smoothie (195 calories)

Dinner – Lentil, Chickpea, and Tomato Soup (291 calories)

Dessert – Coconut, Tahini, and Cashew Bars (155 calories)

Total Calories: 1081 calories

Day 2

Breakfast – Cherry and Walnut Overnight Oats (172 calories)

Lunch – Herby Black Bean Salad with Feta Cheese (245 calories)

Snack – Fish Sticks (238 calories)

Dinner – Grilled Chicken Kabobs (296 calories)

Dessert – Vanilla Baked Pears (216 calories)

Total Calories: 1167 calories

Day 3

Breakfast – Yogurt with Blueberries and Honey (196 calories)

Lunch – Vegetarian Pasta Carbonara (300 calories)

Snack – Orange Salad (186 calories)

Dinner – Italian Minestrone Soup (301.7 calories)

Dessert – Grilled Watermelon Salad (171 calories)

Total Calories: 1154.7 calories

Day 4

Breakfast – Shakshuka (118 calories)

Lunch – Tomato, Basil, and Chickpea Salad (354 calories)

Snack – Trail Mix (218.5 calories)

Dinner – Roasted Tomato and Basil Soup (322 calories)

Dessert – Strawberry Popsicles (38 calories)

Total Calories: 1050.5 calories

Day 5

Breakfast – Greek-Style Frittata (224 calories)

Lunch – Tuna Patties (216 calories)

Snack – Pineapple and Green Smoothie (195 calories)

Dinner – Lentil, Chickpea and Tomato Soup (291 calories)

Dessert – Coconut, Tahini, and Cashew Bars (155 calories)

Total Calories: 1081 calories

Day 6

Breakfast – Cherry and Walnut Overnight Oats (172 calories)

Lunch – Herby Black Bean Salad with Feta Cheese (245 calories)

Snack – Fish Sticks (238 calories)

Dinner – Grilled Chicken Kabobs (296 calories)

Dessert – Vanilla Baked Pears (216 calories)

Total Calories: 1167 calories

Day 7

Breakfast – Yogurt with Blueberries and Honey (196 calories)

Lunch – Vegetarian Pasta Carbonara (300 calories)

Snack – Orange Salad (186 calories)

Dinner – Italian Minestrone Soup (301.7 calories)

Dessert – Grilled Watermelon Salad (171 calories)

Total Calories: 1154.7 calories

Week 2

Day 8

Breakfast – Mini Quiche with Spinach and Mushroom (236 calories)

Lunch – Tabouli Salad (257 calories)

Snack – Chia and Pomegranate Smoothie (208 calories)

Dinner – Cod with Tomatoes and Olives (256 calories)

Dessert – Applesauce Oat Muffins (196 calories)

Total Calories: 1153 calories

Day 9

Breakfast – Quinoa and Chia Oatmeal Mix (162 calories)

Lunch – Mediterranean Cauliflower Pizza (200 calories)

Snack – Kale Chips (176 calories)

Dinner – Greek Turkey Burgers (376 calories)

Dessert – Rice Pudding with Almond Milk (257 calories)

Total Calories: 1171 calories

Day 10

Breakfast – Zucchini with Egg (213 calories)

Lunch – Quinoa and Avocado Salad (236 calories)

Snack – Mediterranean Fruit Salad (201 calories)

Dinner – Greek Pasta (308.3 calories)

Dessert – Watermelon and Mint Granita (168 calories)

Total Calories: 1126.3 calories

Day 11

Breakfast – Breakfast Quinoa with Blueberry and Lemon (269 calories)

Lunch – Mediterranean Salmon (301 calories)

Snack – Tahini and Date Shake (199.4 calories)

Dinner – Shrimp in Garlic Sauce (268.5 calories)

Dessert – Chocolate Dipped Strawberries (235 calories)

Total Calories: 1272.9 calories

Day 12

Breakfast – Mini Quiche with Spinach and Mushroom (236 calories)

Lunch – Tabouli Salad (257 calories)

Snack – Chia and Pomegranate Smoothie (208 calories)

Dinner – Cod with Tomatoes and Olives (256 calories)

Dessert – Applesauce Oat Muffins (196 calories)

Total Calories: 1153 calories

Day 13

Breakfast – Quinoa and Chia Oatmeal Mix (162 calories)

Lunch – Mediterranean Cauliflower Pizza (200 calories)

Snack – Kale Chips (176 calories)

Dinner – Greek Turkey Burgers (376 calories)

Dessert – Rice Pudding with Almond Milk (257 calories)

Total Calories: 1171 calories

Day 14

Breakfast – Zucchini with Egg (213 calories)

Lunch – Quinoa and Avocado Salad (236 calories)

Snack – Mediterranean Fruit Salad (201 calories)

Dinner – Greek Pasta (308.3 calories)

Dessert – Watermelon and Mint Granita (168 calories)

Total Calories: 1126.3 calories

Week 3

Day 15

Breakfast – Spinach and Goat Cheese Quiche (183.1 calories)

Lunch – Chickpea and Quinoa Bowl (273 calories)

Snack – Roasted Chickpeas (208 calories)

Dinner – Hasselback Caprese Chicken (311 calories)

Dessert – Olive Oil Gelato (234 calories)

Total Calories: 1209.1 calories

Day 16

Breakfast – Baked Eggs in Avocado (280 calories)

Lunch – Shrimp Linguine (231 calories)

Snack – Vegetable Chips (100 calories)

Dinner – Greek Red Lentil Soup (293.3 calories)

Dessert – Vanilla Baked Pears (216 calories)

Total Calories: 1120.3 calories

Day 17

Breakfast – Blackberry and Ginger Overnight Bulgur (110 calories)

Lunch – Roasted Eggplants (249.7 calories)

Snack – Flatbread Crackers (190 calories)

Dinner – Grilled Sea Bass (305 calories)

Dessert – Chocolate Avocado Mousse (240 calories)

Total Calories: 1094.7 calories

Day 18

Breakfast – Avocado Toast with Egg (197 calories)

Lunch – Bean Burgers (323.3 calories)

Snack – Baked Zucchini Sticks (132 calories)

Dinner – Sweet and Sour Chicken (375 calories)

Dessert – Baked Apple Slices (228 calories)

Total Calories: 1255.3 calories

Day 19

Breakfast – Spinach and Goat Cheese Quiche (183.1 calories)

Lunch – Chickpea and Quinoa Bowl (273 calories)

Snack – Roasted Chickpeas (208 calories)

Dinner – Hasselback Caprese Chicken (311 calories)

Dessert – Olive Oil Gelato (234 calories)

Total Calories: 1209.1 calories

Day 20

Breakfast – Baked Eggs in Avocado (280 calories)

Lunch – Shrimp Linguine (231 calories)

Snack – Vegetable Chips (100 calories)

Dinner – Greek Red Lentil Soup (293.3 calories)

Dessert – Vanilla Baked Pears (216 calories)

Total Calories: 1120.3 calories

Day 21

Breakfast – Blackberry and Ginger Overnight Bulgur (110 calories)

Lunch – Roasted Eggplants (249.7 calories)

Snack – Flatbread Crackers (190 calories)

Dinner – Grilled Sea Bass (305 calories)

Dessert – Chocolate Avocado Mousse (240 calories)

Total Calories: 1094.7 calories

Week 4

Day 22

Breakfast – Greek-Style Frittata (224 calories)

Lunch – Tuna Patties (216 calories)

Snack – Pineapple and Green Smoothie (195 calories)

Dinner – Lentil, Chickpea and Tomato Soup (291 calories)

Dessert – Coconut, Tahini, and Cashew Bars (155 calories)

Total Calories: 1081 calories

Day 23

Breakfast – Cherry and Walnut Overnight Oats (172 calories)

Lunch – Herby Black Bean Salad with Feta Cheese (245 calories)

Snack – Fish Sticks (238 calories)

Dinner – Grilled Chicken Kabobs (296 calories)

Dessert – Vanilla Baked Pears (216 calories)

Total Calories: 1167 calories

Day 24

Breakfast – Yogurt with Blueberries and Honey (196 calories)

Lunch – Vegetarian Pasta Carbonara (300 calories)

Snack – Orange Salad (186 calories)

Dinner – Italian Minestrone Soup (301.7 calories)

Dessert – Grilled Watermelon Salad (171 calories)

Total Calories: 1154.7 calories

Day 25

Breakfast – Shakshuka (118 calories)

Lunch – Tomato, Basil, and Chickpea Salad (354 calories)

Snack – Trail Mix (218.5 calories)

Dinner – Roasted Tomato and Basil Soup (322 calories)

Dessert – Strawberry Popsicles (38 calories)

Total Calories: 1050.5 calories

Day 26
Breakfast – Greek-Style Frittata (224 calories)
Lunch – Tuna Patties (216 calories)
Snack – Pineapple and Green Smoothie (195 calories)
Dinner – Lentil, Chickpea and Tomato Soup (291 calories)
Dessert – Coconut, Tahini, and Cashew Bars (155 calories)
Total Calories: 1081 calories

Day 27
Breakfast – Cherry and Walnut Overnight Oats (172 calories)
Lunch – Herby Black Bean Salad with Feta Cheese (245 calories)
Snack – Fish Sticks (238 calories)
Dinner – Grilled Chicken Kabobs (296 calories)
Dessert – Vanilla Baked Pears (216 calories)
Total Calories: 1167 calories

Day 28
Breakfast – Yogurt with Blueberries and Honey (196 calories)
Lunch – Vegetarian Pasta Carbonara (300 calories)
Snack – Orange Salad (186 calories)
Dinner – Italian Minestrone Soup (301.7 calories)
Dessert – Grilled Watermelon Salad (171 calories)
Total Calories: 1154.7 calories

Day 29
Breakfast – Mini Quiche with Spinach and Mushroom (236 calories)
Lunch – Tabouli Salad (257 calories)
Snack – Chia and Pomegranate Smoothie (208 calories)

Dinner – Cod with Tomatoes and Olives (256 calories)
Dessert – Applesauce Oat Muffins (196 calories)
Total Calories: 1153 calories

Day 30
Breakfast – Quinoa and Chia Oatmeal Mix (162 calories)
Lunch – Mediterranean Cauliflower Pizza (200 calories)
Snack – Kale Chips (176 calories)
Dinner – Greek Turkey Burgers (376 calories)

Dessert – Rice Pudding with Almond Milk (257 calories)
Total Calories: 1171 calories

Meal Prep Tips

Save time by spending Sunday or any day of the week to prepare the meals for the week ahead. I have always started with making the ingredients lists and checking which foods are present in my pantry and what I need to buy. Meal prep containers for meals, meal prep jars for salad and smoothies, plastic bags, and aluminum foil would greatly help you pack each serving for you and your family members. Some stickers would also be required to label the meals.

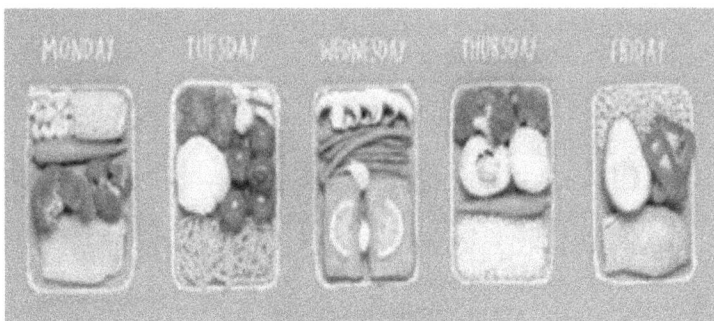

For Meals (breakfast, lunch, snack, dinner, and dessert): When you are done cooking the meals, cool them at room temperature, divide them evenly in meal prep containers and keep them in the refrigerator. When ready to eat, let the meals rest at room temperature for 5 to 10 minutes and then microwave for 1 to 2 minutes at a high heat setting until thoroughly warmed.

You can also pack servings of muffins, frittata, and quiche in just aluminum foil. Prepare oats dishes in the meal prep containers, keep them in the refrigerator and just stir.

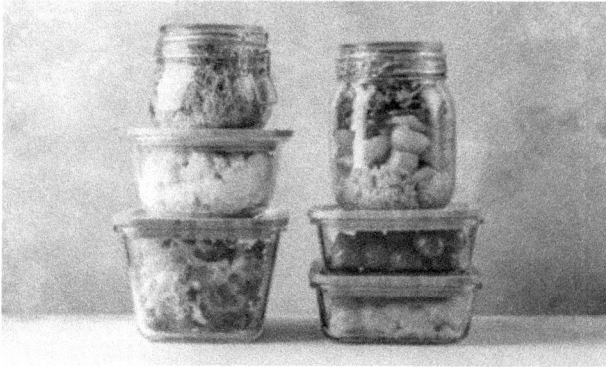

For Salads: Spoon the prepared salad dressing in the bottom of a salad jar, add beans, grains, or hard vegetables such as cucumber, layer with soft vegetables such as avocado and tomatoes, top with proteins, and then layer it with leafy greens of the salad. When ready to eat, mix the salad within the jar until the ingredients have been coated in the salad dressing.

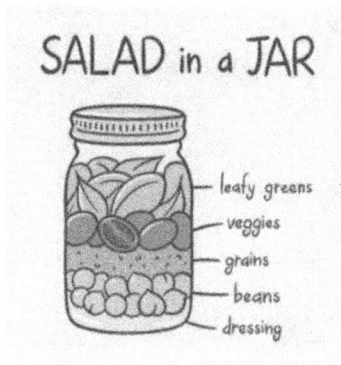

For Smoothie:

Add all the solid ingredients in an 8-ounce mason jar or a large plastic bag, seal it, and keep it in the refrigerator until required. When ready to drink, transfer the smoothie ingredients for its bag to a blender, add the liquid and then pulse until smooth. If you have your ingredients in a mason jar, then just pour in the liquid and blend the ingredients with an immersion blender.

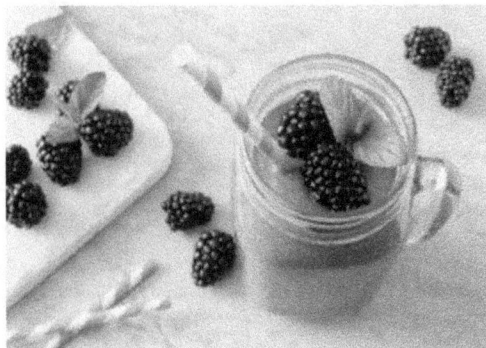

For Sauces, Dips, and Dressings:

Spoon the prepared sauces, dips, and dressing in 4 to 8 ounces mason jars; cover with a thin film of oil to prevent oxidation. Seal the mason jars with their lids and store them in the refrigerator. Try to use sauces, dips, and dressing as fresh and avoid freezing them.

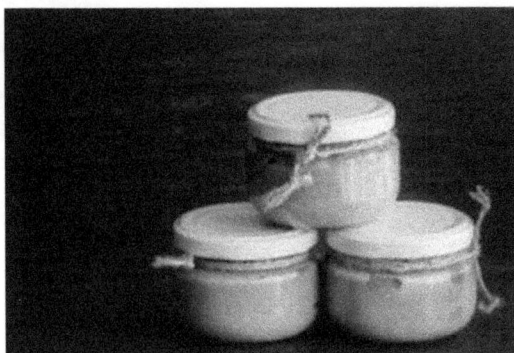

For Snacks:

Like the meal, cool the cooked snacks, divide them in even portions among the meal prep containers or plastic bags, seal them, and keep them in the refrigerator. For snacks such as fruit salad, you can also pack it straight away in the meal prep container. Pack solid snacks such as crackers and chickpeas in a plastic bag.

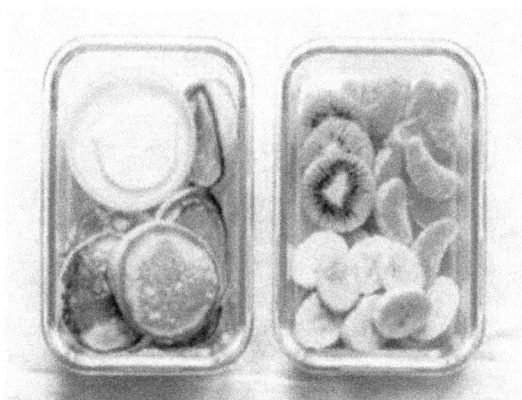

Make sure you label the meal prep containers, jars, and plastic bags with the recipe name and day to eat them.

Chapter 5

Sauces, Dips, and Dressings

Tzatziki Sauce

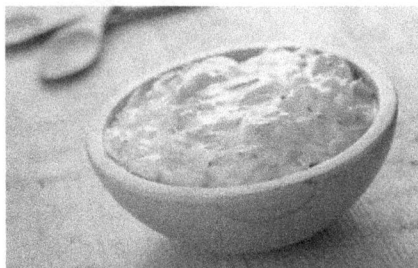

Nutritional Information per Serving

Calories: 28 calories
Fat: 1.9g
Sat. Fat: 0.6g
Carbohydrates: 1.6g
Protein: 0.9g
Fiber: 0.1g

Prep Time: 15 minutes | Cook Time: 0 minutes | Servings: ½ cup; 1 tablespoon per serving
Ingredients

- 1 teaspoon minced garlic
- ½ of a medium cucumber, peeled, grated
- 1/8 teaspoon salt, and more as needed for cucumber
- ¼ teaspoon dried dill
- ¾ tablespoon olive oil
- ½ cup yogurt, low-fat

Directions

- Place the grated cucumber in a colander, sprinkle salt on it, and let it sit for 10 minutes.
- Then squeeze the excess water out from the cucumber, and transfer it to a large bowl.
- Add yogurt, oil, garlic, dill, and ⅛ teaspoon salt, into the bowl, and stir until combined.
- Then cover the bowl with its lid, place it in the refrigerator and let it rest for 30 minutes or more until required and ready to serve.
- **Storing Option:** For storing the sauce, transfer it to an air-tight container and keep it in the refrigerator for up to 1 week; don't freeze it.

Tahini Sauce

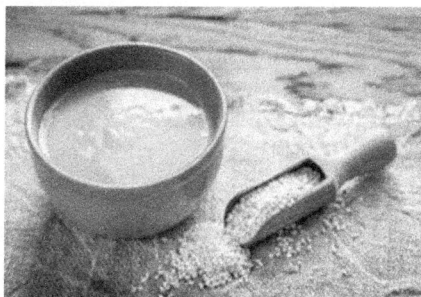

Nutritional Information per Serving

Calories: 124 calories
Fat: 10.8g
Sat. Fat: 1.5g
Carbohydrates: 5.6g
Protein: 3.6g
Fiber: 1.9g

Prep Time: 15 minutes | Cook Time: 0 minutes | Servings: 1 cup; 3 tablespoons per serving

Ingredients

- 4 medium cloves of garlic, peeled, minced
- 1/8 teaspoon ground cumin
- ¼ cup lemon juice
- ½ teaspoon sea salt
- ½ cup tahini
- 6 tablespoons of water, ice-chilled

Directions

- Take a medium bowl, place garlic in it, add lemon juice, stir until well mixed and then let the mixture rest for 10 minutes.
- Take a separate medium bowl, place a fine-mesh sieve on it and then pass the lemon-garlic mixture through it, pressing garlic with the back of a spoon or spatula to extract liquid as much as possible.
- Add tahini into the collected liquid along with cumin and salt, and then whisk. until blended.
- Then whisk 2 tablespoons of water at a time until smooth and creamy sauce comes together, and then store the sauce in an air-tight jar.
- Storing Option: Keep the sauce in the refrigerator for up to 1 week or freeze it for up to 1 month.

Pesto Genovese

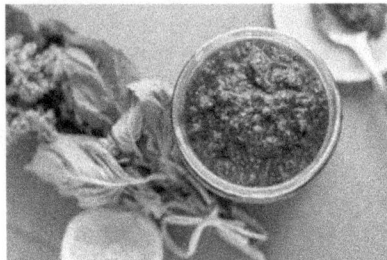

Nutritional Information per Serving

Calories: 123 calories
Fat: 11.5g
Sat. Fat: 3.1g
Carbohydrates: 1.9g
Protein: 3.8g
Fiber: 0.4g

Prep Time: 10 minutes | Cook Time: 0 minutes | Servings: 1 cup; 1 tablespoon per serving

Ingredients

- 2 ounces basil leaves, washed
- 1 clove of garlic, peeled
- 3 tablespoons pine nuts
- ¼ teaspoon salt
- 3 tablespoons Pecorino Sardo cheese, low-fat
- ¼ cup olive oil
- ½ cup parmesan cheese, low-fat

Directions

- Plug in a food processor, add pecorino cheese, parmesan, garlic, pine nuts, salt, and basil leaves.
- Pulse until the mixture turns smooth, and then slowly blend in oil until combined.
- When done, spoon the prepared pesto mixture into a serving bowl, and serve.
- Storing Option: For storing the pesto sauce, transfer it to an air-tight container and keep it in the refrigerator for up to 1 week or freeze it for up to 1 month.

Italian Red Pesto

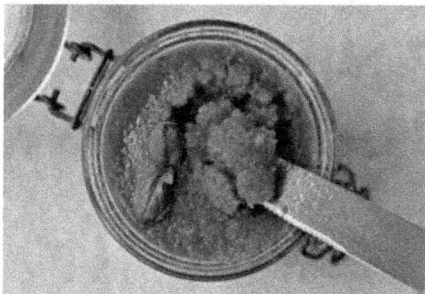

Nutritional Information per Serving

Calories: 91.8 calories
Fat: 8.6g
Sat. Fat: 1.5g
Carbohydrates: 2.06g
Protein: 1.3g
Fiber: 0.5g

Prep Time: 10 minutes | Cook Time: 0 minutes | Servings: ½ cup; 1 tablespoon per serving

Ingredients

- 3 tablespoons almonds
- ½ cup arugula, packed
- ¼ cup sun-dried tomatoes, diced
- 1 clove of garlic, peeled
- 2 tablespoons ricotta cheese, low-fat
- ¼ cup olive oil
- 2 tablespoons grated parmesan cheese, low-fat

Directions

- Plug in a food processor, add garlic, almonds, and tomatoes, and then pulse until chunky.
- Then add arugula, and parmesan, pulse until just mixed, and slowly blend in oil until combined.
- When done, spoon the prepared pesto mixture into a bowl, and serve.

- **Storing Option:** For storing the pesto sauce, transfer it to an air-tight container and keep it in the refrigerator for up to 1 week or freeze it for up to 1 month.

Salsa Verde

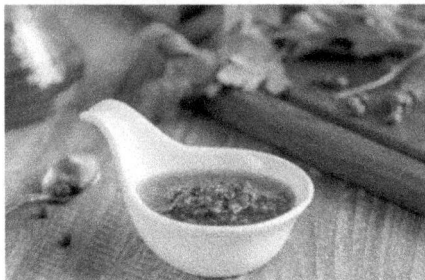

Nutritional Information per Serving

Calories: 48 calories
Fat: 5g
Sat. Fat: 0.7g
Carbohydrates: 0.6g
Protein: 0.6g
Fiber: 0.2g

Prep Time: 10 minutes | Cook Time: 0 minutes | Servings: ½ cup; 1 tablespoon per serving

Ingredients

- ¾ cup parsley, minced
- ½ teaspoon minced garlic
- ¾ tablespoon minced capers
- ¼ teaspoon red chili flakes
- ¼ teaspoon salt
- ¼ teaspoon crushed black pepper
- 3 tablespoons olive oil
- 1 teaspoon lemon juice
- ½ teaspoon lemon zest

Directions

- Take a medium bowl, place parsley in it, add capers and garlic, and stir until mixed.

- Then add lemon zest, lemon juice, salt, red chili flakes, black pepper, and oil, and then stir until mixed and well combined.
- When done, spoon the salsa mixture into a serving bowl, and serve.
- Storing Option: For storing the salsa, transfer it to an air-tight container and keep it in the refrigerator for up to 1 week or freeze it for up to 1 month.

Baba Ganoush

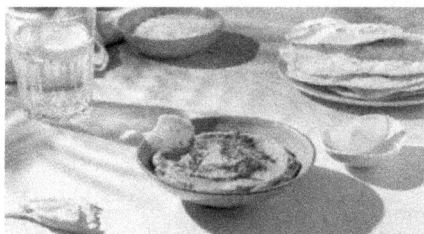

Nutritional Information per Serving

Calories: 27.9 calories
Fat: 1.9g
Sat. Fat: 0.2g
Carbohydrates: 2.2g
Protein: 0.3g
Fiber: 1.1g

Prep Time: 10 minutes | Cook Time: 20 minutes | Servings: 1 cup; 1 tablespoon per serving

Ingredients

- 1 medium eggplant
- 1 clove of garlic, peeled
- ½ teaspoon sumac
- ¼ teaspoon salt
- ¼ teaspoon ground black pepper

- ½ teaspoon cayenne pepper
- 1 ½ tablespoon tahini sauce
- 2 tablespoons olive oil
- 1 tablespoon lemon juice

Directions

- Switch on the oven, then set it to 218 degrees C or 425 degrees F, and preheat.
- Meanwhile, take a baking tray, grease it with cooking spray, and set it aside until required.
- Place the eggplant on a cutting board, slice it in half, and then make a few slits on the skin of the eggplant.
- Sprinkle the eggplant halves with salt, rub it well on the skin of the eggplant, let it sit for 10 minutes, and then wipe it with a cloth dry.
- Place the eggplant skin-side-down on the prepared baking tray, drizzle with oil on top, and then bake for 20 to 30 minutes, or until soft.

- When done, transfer the baked eggplant to a plate, set it aside to cool at room temperature, spoon the insides of the eggplant, and transfer to a food processor.

- Add yogurt, tahini, garlic, lime juice, cayenne, salt, black pepper, and sumac, and pulse until smooth and combined.
- Spoon the dip into a bowl, cover the bowl with its lid, place it into the refrigerator, let it rest for 30 minutes and then serve.
- Storing Option: For storing the baba ganoush, transfer it to an air-tight container and keep it in the refrigerator for up to 5 days; don't freeze it.

Lebanese Hummus

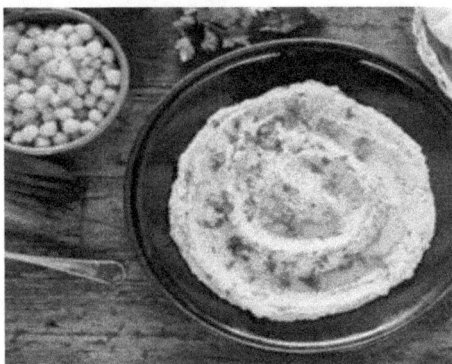

Nutritional Information per Serving

Calories: 152 calories
Fat: 15g
Sat. Fat: 2g
Carbohydrates: 5g
Protein: 2g
Fiber: 1g

Prep Time: 10 minutes | Cook Time: 0 minutes | Servings: 1 cup; 1 tablespoon per serving

Ingredients

- 10 ounces chickpeas, canned, drained, rinsed
- 1 teaspoon minced garlic
- 1 teaspoon crushed pine nuts
- ¼ teaspoon paprika

- 2 tablespoons tahini sauce
- ¼ teaspoon salt
- 2 tablespoons olive oil
- 2 tablespoons lemon juice
- 2 tablespoons water

Directions

- Plug in a food processor, add garlic, chickpeas, paprika, salt, tahini, lemon juice, oil, and water, and pulse until smooth and blended.

- When done, spoon the prepared hummus into a serving bowl, sprinkle pine nuts on top, and serve.
- Storing Option: For storing the hummus, transfer it to an air-tight container and keep it in the refrigerator for up to 1 week or freeze it for up to 1 month.

Guacamole

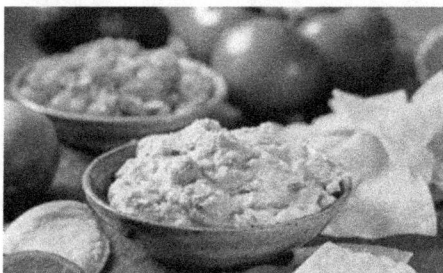

Nutritional Information per Serving

Calories: 44.3 calories
Fat: 2.4g
Sat. Fat: 0.2g
Carbohydrates: 4.4g
Protein: 1.2g
Fiber: 1.1g

Prep Time: 10 minutes | Cook Time: 0 minutes | Servings: 1 cup; 1 tablespoon per serving

Ingredients

- 1 small white onion, peeled, chopped
- 2 medium avocados, halved, pitted
- ½ of a medium tomato, chopped
- ½ of medium green bell pepper, cored, chopped
- 2 tablespoons chopped cilantro, fresh
- ¼ teaspoon salt
- 1 teaspoon olive oil
- 2 tablespoons lemon juice

Directions

- Place the avocados on a cutting board, cut it in half, remove the pit and then spoon the insides of the avocados into a large bowl.
- Take a fork to mash the avocados in the bowl, and then add cilantro, tomato, onion, bell pepper, salt, lemon juice, and oil.
- Stir until combined and well mixed, then spoon the prepared mixture into a serving bowl, and serve.

- **Storing Option:** For storing the guacamole, spoon it into an air-tight container, smooth the top, cover it with a thin layer of lemon juice, shut the container tightly with its lid, and refrigerate for up to 1 week; don't freeze it.

Roasted Tomato Spread (Matbucha)

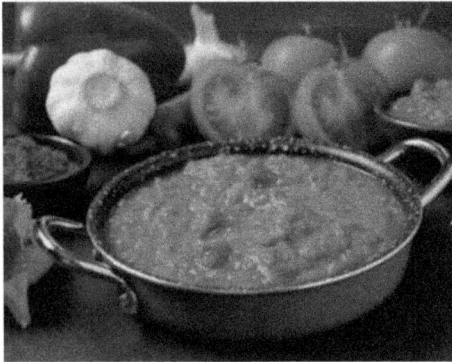

Nutritional Information per Serving

Calories: 27.5 calories
Fat: 1.7g
Sat. Fat: 0.2g
Carbohydrates: 2.6g
Protein: 0.3g
Fiber: 0.7g

Prep Time: 10 minutes | Cook Time: 20 minutes | Servings: 1 cup; 1 tablespoon per serving

Ingredients

- 4 small tomatoes, halved
- 1 large green bell pepper, quartered
- 3 cloves of garlic, peeled
- 2 tablespoons cilantro leaves
- 1 large white onion, peeled, quartered
- 2 tablespoons parsley leaves
- ¼ teaspoon salt
- 1 teaspoon red chili flakes
- ¼ teaspoon ground black pepper
- 1 tablespoon lemon juice
- 2 tablespoons olive oil, divided

Directions

- Switch on the oven, then set it to 190 degrees C or 347 degrees F, and preheat.
- Meanwhile, take a baking tray, grease it with cooking spray, and set it aside.

- Take a large bowl, place tomatoes, green peppers, onions, and garlic in it, add 1 tablespoon oil, salt, red pepper flakes, and black pepper, and toss until well mixed.
- Transfer the vegetables to the prepared baking tray and spread them in a single layer.
- Place the tray in the oven and bake for 20 to 30 minutes, or until golden brown.
- When done, let the vegetables cool at room temperature and then transfer them into a food processor.
- Add remaining oil along with parsley and cilantro, pulse until the mixture is combined and chunky, spoon the dip into a bowl and then serve.
- **Storing Option:** For storing the spread, transfer it to an air-tight container and keep it in the refrigerator for up to 1 week or freeze it for up to 1 month.

Pickled Mango Sauce

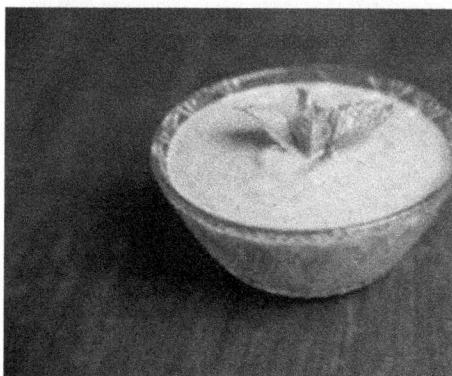

Nutritional Information per Serving

Calories: 27.8 calories
Fat: 1.7g
Sat. Fat: 0.2g
Carbohydrates: 2.7g
Protein: 0.2g
Fiber: 0.4g

Prep Time: 15 minutes | Cook Time: 8 minutes | Servings: 1 ½ cups; 1 tablespoon per serving

Ingredients

- 1 large mango, peeled, cut into
- ½ teaspoon ground coriander

- chunks
- ½ teaspoon minced garlic
- 1 tablespoon coconut sugar
- ¾ tablespoon salt
- ½ teaspoon mustard seeds
- ½ teaspoon ground fenugreek
- 1 teaspoon cumin seeds

- ½ teaspoon turmeric powder
- ½ teaspoon ground black pepper
- 1 tablespoon paprika
- 3 tablespoons olive oil
- ½ cup water

Directions

- Place the mango chunks on a cutting board, sprinkle with salt, transfer into a glass jar, close with its lid and let the jar rest in the sun for 5 days.
- Then drain the excess water out from the jar, spread the mango chunks on parchment paper, and let them dry for 4 hours.
- Take a small pot, place it over low heat, add mustard seed, fenugreek, cumin, coriander, turmeric, black pepper, paprika.
- Stir while cooking for 3 minutes, add coconut sugar and garlic, cook for 3 minutes, add mangoes and water and then stir until well combined.
- Then plug in a blender, add the prepared mango mixture, pulse until smooth, and serve.
- Storing Option: For storing the sauce, transfer it to an air-tight container and keep it in the refrigerator for up to 1 week; don't freeze it.

Cherry Tomato Sauce

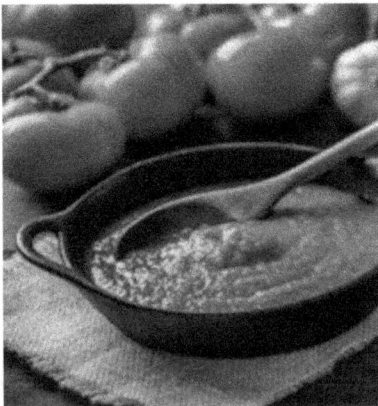

Nutritional Information per Serving

Calories: 21 calories
Fat: 1.7g
Sat. Fat: 0.2g
Carbohydrates: 1.1g
Protein: 0.2g
Fiber: 0.2g

Prep Time: 10 minutes | Cook Time: 20 minutes | Servings: 2 cups; 1 tablespoon per serving

Ingredients

- 1 quart of cherry tomatoes, stems removed
- 1 teaspoon minced garlic
- ½ teaspoon dried oregano
- ¼ teaspoon salt
- ¼ teaspoon ground black pepper
- ¼ cup olive oil
- 2 tablespoons balsamic vinegar

Directions

- Switch on the oven, then set it to 204 degrees C or 400 degrees F, and preheat.
- Meanwhile, take a baking tray, grease it with cooking spray, and set it aside until required.
- Scatter the cherry tomatoes on the prepared baking tray in a single layer, drizzle with oil and balsamic vinegar, and then sprinkle salt, black pepper, oregano, and garlic.
- Bake the tomatoes for 20 minutes, or until soft, let the tomatoes cool at room temperature and transfer into a blender.
- Pulse the tomato mixture until smooth, and then serve.
- Storing Option: For storing the sauce, transfer it to an air-tight container and keep it in the refrigerator for up to 1 week or freeze it for up to 1 month.

Roasted Red Pepper Dip (Muhammara)

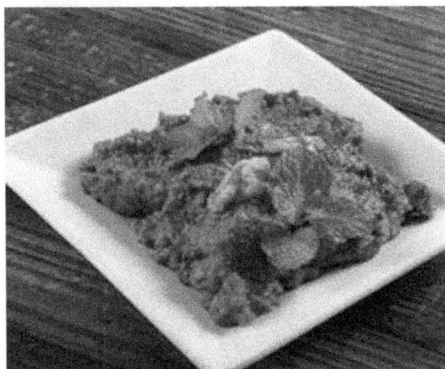

Nutritional Information per Serving

Calories: 54 calories
Fat: 4.7g
Sat. Fat: 0.6g
Carbohydrates: 2.1g
Protein: 0.6g
Fiber: 0.4g

Prep Time: 10 minutes | Cook Time: 20 minutes | Servings: 1 cup; 1 tablespoon per serving

Ingredients

- ½ cup walnuts, roasted
- 1 medium bell pepper, halved, roasted
- 1 clove of garlic, peeled
- 2 tablespoons whole-wheat breadcrumbs
- ½ teaspoon salt
- ¼ teaspoon crushed red pepper flakes
- ½ teaspoon ground cumin
- 3 tablespoons olive oil
- ½ teaspoon pomegranate molasses
- ½ tablespoon lemon juice

Directions

- Plug in a blender, add roasted bell pepper, roasted walnuts, oil, salt, cumin, red pepper, and breadcrumbs.
- Add garlic, molasses, and lemon juice, pulse until smooth and well combined.
- When done, spoon the prepared mixture into a serving bowl, and serve.
- Storing Option: For storing the dip, transfer it to an air-tight container and keep it in the refrigerator for up to 1 week; don't freeze it.

Ranch Dressing

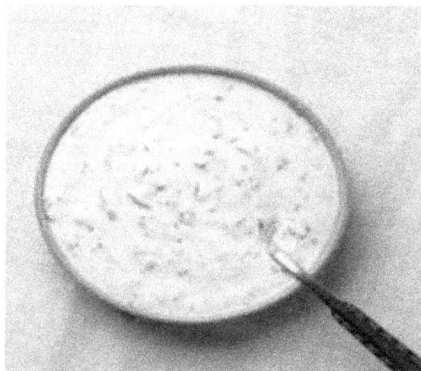

Nutritional Information per Serving

Calories: 52.7 calories
Fat: 5.5g
Sat. Fat: 0.9g
Carbohydrates: 0.9g
Protein: 0.4g
Fiber: 0.01g

Prep Time: 10 minutes | Cook Time: 10 minutes | Servings: 1 cup; 1 tablespoon per serving

Ingredients

- ½ tablespoon parsley
- ½ tablespoon dill
- ½ tablespoon onion powder
- ½ tablespoon garlic powder
- ¼ teaspoon salt
- ¼ teaspoon ground black pepper
- ½ tablespoon apple cider vinegar
- ¼ cup yogurt, low-fat
- ½ cup mayonnaise, low-fat

Directions

- Take a large mixing bowl, place mayonnaise, yogurt, and vinegar in it, and whisk until well combined.
- Add onion powder, garlic powder, salt, black pepper, dill, parsley, and whisk until well mixed and smooth.
- When done, spoon the prepared dressing into a serving bowl, and serve.
- Storing Option: For storing the dressing, transfer it to an air-tight container and keep it in the refrigerator for up to 5 days; don't freeze it.

Tangy Italian Salad Dressing

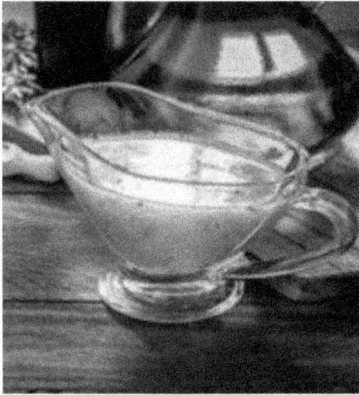

Nutritional Information per Serving

Calories: 81.1 calories
Fat: 8.5g
Sat. Fat: 1.2g
Carbohydrates: 0.6g
Protein: 0.6g
Fiber: 0.6g

Prep Time: 5 minutes | Cook Time: 0 minutes | Servings: ½ cup; 1 tablespoon per serving

Ingredients

- 1 teaspoon minced garlic
- ¼ teaspoon dried oregano
- ¼ teaspoon dried basil
- ¼ teaspoon salt
- ⅓ cup olive oil
- ¼ teaspoon whole-grain mustard
- 3 tablespoons red wine vinegar
- 1 tablespoon lemon juice

Directions

- Take a large jar, add garlic, basil, oregano, salt, and add mustard, oil, vinegar, and lemon juice.
- Cover the jar with its lid and then shake it well until combined and mixed.
- When done, spoon the prepared dressing into a serving bowl, and serve.
- Storing Option: For storing the dressing, transfer it to an air-tight container and keep it in the refrigerator for up to 5 days; don't freeze it.

Yogurt Tahini Dressing

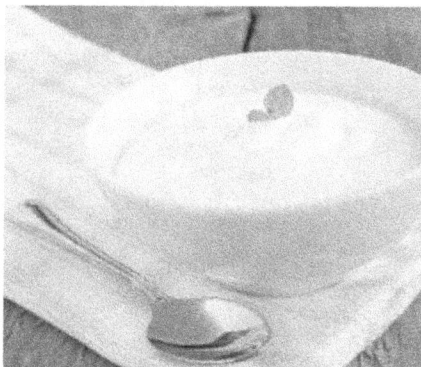

Nutritional Information per Serving

Calories: 27 calories
Fat: 1.5g
Sat. Fat: 0.7g
Carbohydrates: 1.8g
Protein: 1.3g
Fiber: 0.1g

Prep Time: 5 minutes | Cook Time: 0 minutes | Servings: 1 cup; 1 tablespoon per serving

Ingredients

- ½ teaspoon minced garlic
- ¼ teaspoon salt
- 2 tablespoons lemon juice
- 2 teaspoons tahini
- 1 cup yogurt, low-fat
- ½ teaspoon lemon zest

Directions

- Take a medium bowl, place yogurt and tahini in it, add salt, garlic, lemon juice, and lemon zest, and stir until well combined.
- When done, spoon the prepared dressing into a serving bowl, and serve.
- Storing Option: For storing the dressing, transfer it to an air-tight container and keep it in the refrigerator for up to 5 days; don't freeze it.

Balsamic, Dill and Yogurt Dressing

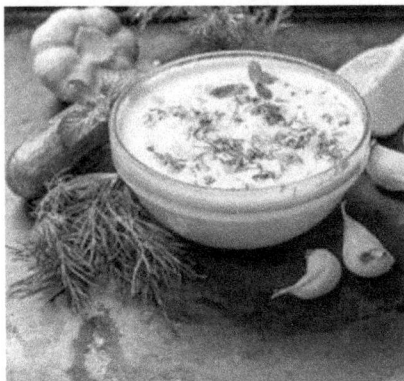

Nutritional Information per Serving

Calories: 67 calories
Fat: 6.9g
Sat. Fat: 1.1g
Carbohydrates: 0.5g
Protein: 0.5g
Fiber: 0.05g

Prep Time: 5 minutes | Cook Time: 0 minutes | Servings: ½ cup; 1 tablespoon per serving

Ingredients

- 1 teaspoon minced garlic
- ¼ teaspoon salt
- ¼ teaspoon dried oregano
- ¼ teaspoon dried dill
- ¼ cup olive oil
- ½ tablespoon whole-grain mustard
- ¼ cup yogurt, low-fat
- 2 tablespoons apple cider vinegar

Directions

- Take a medium bowl, place garlic, yogurt, and vinegar in it, add salt, oregano, dill, mustard, and whisk until well combined.
- Then gently whisk in oil until incorporated, and smooth, and then serve.
- Storing Option: For storing the dressing, transfer it to an air-tight container and keep it in the refrigerator for up to 5 days; don't freeze it.

Chapter 6

Breakfast

Greek-Style Frittata

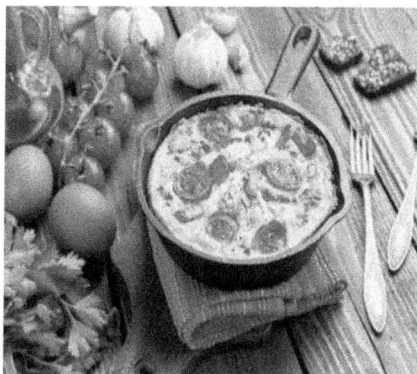

Nutritional Information per Serving

Calories: 224 calories
Fat: 15g
Sat. Fat: 4g
Carbohydrates: 7g
Protein: 15g
Fiber: 2g

Prep Time: 10 minutes | Cook Time: 12 minutes | Servings: 1 Frittata, 1 slice per serving

Ingredients

- ½ cup dried tomato slices, not oil-packed
- 6 tablespoons Italian marinated olive antipasto
- 1 teaspoon dried oregano, crushed
- ½ cup roasted red sweet peppers, chopped
- ¼ teaspoon ground black pepper
- 8 large eggs, at room temperature
- 2 tablespoons olive oil
- ½ cup boiling water
- 4 tablespoons crumbled feta cheese, reduced-fat
- 1 tablespoon chopped oregano

Directions

- Switch on the oven, then set it to 425 degrees F and let it preheat.
- Meanwhile, take a small bowl, place dried tomatoes in it, pour in the boiling water, stir until just mixed and let the tomatoes stand for 5 minutes.
- In the meantime, take a large bowl, crack eggs in it and then whisk until blended.
- Add dried oregano, red pepper, olive antipasto, and cheese and stir until just mixed.
- Drain the soaked tomatoes, reserving their liquid, and then stir this liquid into the prepared egg mixture.
- Take a large heat-proof skillet pan, place it over medium heat, add oil, and when hot, pour in the egg mixture and then spread it evenly.
- Scatter the soak tomato slices on top, cook for 3 to 4 minutes until the bottom begins to set, and then transfer the skillet pan into the oven.
- Continue cooking the frittata for 5 to 8 minutes until thoroughly cooked and top turn golden.
- When done, slide the frittata into a plate, let it rest for 5 minutes and then cut it into four slices.
- Sprinkle chopped oregano over the frittata slices and then serve.

Spinach and Goat Cheese Quiche

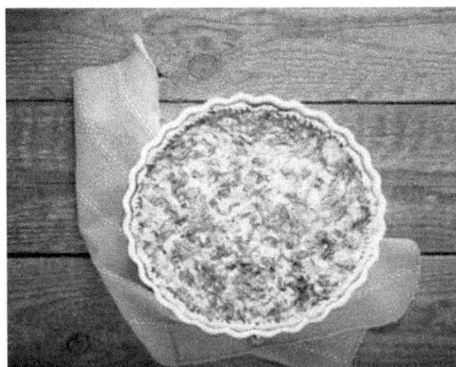

Nutritional Information per Serving

Calories: 183.1 calories
Fat: 10.7g
Sat. Fat: 4.1g
Carbohydrates: 13g
Protein: 9.8g
Fiber: 0.8g

Prep Time: 10 minutes | Cook Time: 30 minutes | Servings: 1 Quiche, 1 slice per serving

Ingredients

- 6 ounces spinach leaves, fresh, chopped
- 1 frozen pie crust, whole-grain, thawed
- 2 medium eggs, at room temperature
- ¼ teaspoon salt
- 1/3 cup half-and-half
- ¼ teaspoon ground black pepper
- 4 slices of goat cheese, fresh, low-fat
- ¼ cup water
- 2 tablespoons sour cream, low-fat

Directions

- Switch on the oven, then set it to 390 degrees F and let it preheat.
- Meanwhile, take a medium skillet pan, place it over medium heat, pour in the water, and then bring it to a simmer.
- Add spinach leaves, cook them for 3 to 4 minutes until leaves have wilted, drain them and then squeeze well to remove excess water.
- Take a medium bowl, crack eggs in it, whisk until blended and then whisk in salt, half-and-half, black pepper, and sour cream until smooth.
- Add the cooked spinach into the egg mixture and then stir until just mixed.
- Place the pie crust into a greased pie pan, fill it with the prepared egg mixture, smooth the top and then scatter the goat cheese slices on top.
- Place the prepared pie pan into the oven and then bake for 20 to 30 minutes until the quiche has set and the top turns golden brown.
- When done, let the quiche in its pan for 5 minutes, then transfer it to a cutting board, cut it into four slices and serve.

Mini Quiche with Spinach and Mushroom

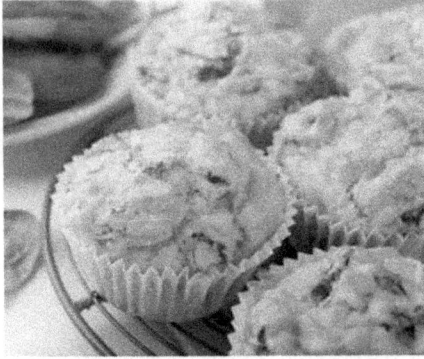

Nutritional Information per Serving

Calories: 236 calories
Fat: 16.4g
Sat. Fat: 5.8g
Carbohydrates: 7.1g
Protein: 15.5g
Fiber: 1.5g

Prep Time: 10 minutes | Cook Time: 30 minutes | Servings: 6 mini-quiche; 2 quiches per serving

Ingredients

- 2 ounces spinach leaves, fresh, chopped
- 4 ounces shiitake mushrooms, sliced
- ½ cup sliced white onion
- ½ tablespoon minced garlic
- 1 teaspoon minced thyme
- ¼ teaspoon salt
- 1 teaspoon whole-grain mustard
- ¼ teaspoon ground black pepper
- 1 tablespoon olive oil
- 4 medium eggs, at room temperature
- 6 tablespoons coconut milk, unsweetened, low-fat
- 6 tablespoons shredded Gruyere or parmesan cheese, low-fat

Directions

- Switch on the oven, then set it to 325 degrees F and let it preheat.
- Meanwhile, take a medium skillet pan, place it over medium heat, add oil and when hot, add mushrooms.
- Spread the mushrooms in a single layer and then cook for 4 minutes per side until brown.

- Then add onion, cook for 2 minutes until softened, stir in garlic and thyme and continue cooking for 2 minutes.
- Add spinach, stir until just mixed, cook for 2 minutes and then remove the pan from heat.
- Take a medium bowl, crack the eggs in it, add salt, black pepper, and mustard, pour in the mustard, and then whisk until blended.
- Add the mushroom mixture along with cheese and then stir until just mixed.
- Take 6 silicone muffin cups, grease them with oil, evenly fill them with the prepared mushroom mixture and then bake for 15 to 20 minutes until thoroughly cooked and firm.
- When done, let the quiche rest in the muffin cups for 5 minutes and then serve.

Baked Eggs in Avocado

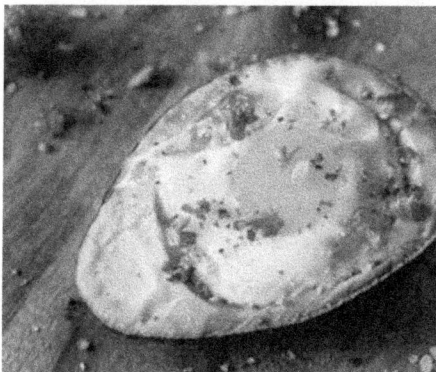

Nutritional Information per Serving

Calories: 280 calories
Fat: 23.5g
Sat. Fat: 4.9g
Carbohydrates: 9.3g
Protein: 11.3g
Fiber: 6.9g

Prep Time: 10 minutes | Cook Time: 15 minutes | Servings: 2; 1 avocado half per serving

Ingredients

- 1 avocado, halved, pitted
- 2 teaspoons chopped chives, fresh
- ¼ teaspoon sea salt
- ¼ teaspoon dried parsley
- ¼ teaspoon ground black pepper
- 2 small eggs, at room temperature

Directions

- Switch on the oven, then set it to 425 degrees F and let it preheat.
- Meanwhile, take a medium bowl and crack the eggs in it, keeping the yolk intact.
- Take a baking dish, arrange avocado halves in it cut-side-up and then spoon an egg yolk into each half.
- Then divide the egg white evenly between the avocado halves and then season with salt, black pepper, chives, and parsley.
- Place the prepared baking dish containing avocado halves into the oven and then bake for 15 minutes or until the eggs have cooked to the desired level.
- Serve straight away.

Avocado Toast with Egg

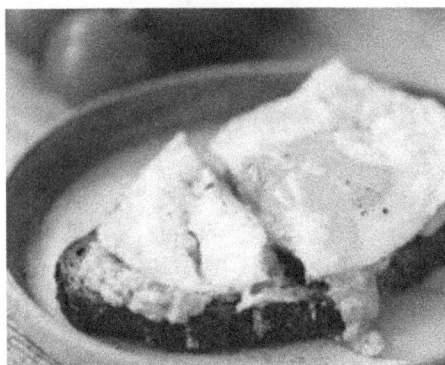

Nutritional Information per Serving

Calories: 197 calories
Fat: 17g
Sat. Fat: 6g
Carbohydrates: 5g
Protein: 7g
Fiber: 3g

Prep Time: 10 minutes | Cook Time: 10 minutes | Servings: 4; 1 toast per serving

Ingredients

- 4 slices of whole-wheat bread
- 1 avocado, peeled, pitted, sliced
- ¼ teaspoon sea salt
- 4 tablespoons butter, low-fat
- ¼ teaspoon ground black pepper
- 4 eggs, at room temperature

Directions

- Prepare the bread slices and for this, toast them until golden and crispy to the desired level.
- Meanwhile, take a medium bowl, place avocado slices in it and then mash with a fork.
- Fry the egg, and for this, take a medium skillet pan, place it over medium heat, add 1 tablespoon butter and when it melts, crack the egg in it and then cook for 5 to 7 minutes until cooked to the desired level.
- Assemble the toast and for this, spread ¼ of the mashed avocado over the toast, sprinkle some salt and black pepper over the top and then top with a fried egg.
- Serve straight away.

Zucchini with Egg

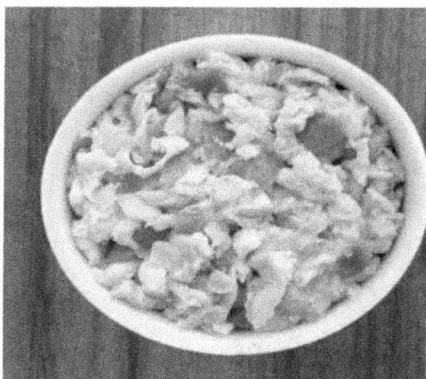

Nutritional Information per Serving

Calories: 213 calories
Fat: 15.7g
Sat. Fat: 3.1g
Carbohydrates: 11.2g
Protein: 10.2g
Fiber: 3.6g

Prep Time: 5 minutes | Cook Time: 18 minutes | Servings: 2; 1 plate per serving

Ingredients

- 2 large zucchinis, ends trimmed, diced
- ½ teaspoon salt
- 1 ½ tablespoon olive oil
- ¼ teaspoon ground black pepper
- 1 teaspoon water
- 2 large eggs, at room temperature

Directions

- Take a medium skillet pan, place it over medium-high heat, add oil and when hot, add zucchini and then cook for 10 minutes until tender.
- Stir salt and black pepper into the zucchini and continue cooking for 1 minute.
- Take a medium bowl, crack the eggs in it, add water and then whisk until blended.
- Pour the blended eggs over the cooked zucchini and then cook for 5 minutes until eggs have scrambled to the desired level.
- Taste the scrambled eggs to adjust seasonings, divide evenly between two plates, and then serve.

Shakshuka

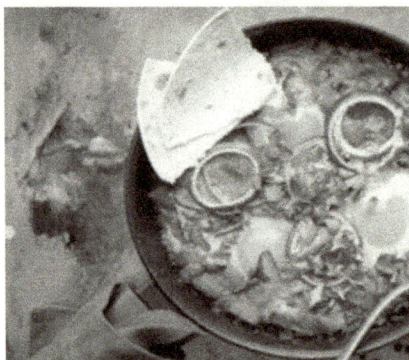

Nutritional Information per Serving

Calories: 118 calories
Fat: 9g
Sat. Fat: 2g
Carbohydrates: 4g
Protein: 7g
Fiber: 1g

Prep Time: 5 minutes | Cook Time: 18 minutes | Servings: 4; 1 egg with tomato mixture per serving

Ingredients

- ½ medium white onion, peeled, chopped
- ½-pound tomatoes, halved
- ¼ cup baby spinach, chopped
- ¼ teaspoon minced garlic
- 1 tablespoon olive oil
- ¼ teaspoon ground pepper
- ½ teaspoon ground cumin
- 4 large eggs, at room temperature

- ¼ teaspoon salt

Directions

- Switch on the oven, then set it to 400 degrees F and let it preheat.
- Meanwhile, take a large heat-proof skillet pan, place it over medium-high heat, add oil, and when hot, add onion and then cook for 4 minutes until golden brown.
- Add salt, black pepper, cumin, and garlic, stir until mixed, and then continue cooking for 1 minute.
- Add tomato halves, stir until just mixed, then transfer the pan into the oven and continue cooking for 5 minutes until tomatoes have roasted.
- When done, stir the tomatoes well, make four small spaces in the tomato mixture and then carefully crack an egg into each space.
- Return the pan into the oven and continue cooking for 3 to 5 minutes until egg yolks turn runny.
- When done, sprinkle spinach over the eggs and then serve with toasted slices of whole-wheat baguette.

Cherry and Walnut Overnight Oats

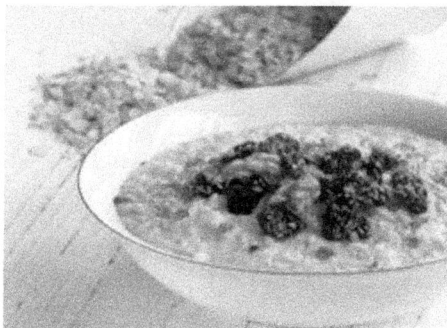

Nutritional Information per Serving

Calories: 162 calories
Fat: 6.2g
Sat. Fat: 1.8g
Carbohydrates: 23g
Protein: 4.3g
Fiber: 2.5g

Prep Time: 8 hours and 10 minutes | Cook Time: 0 minutes | Servings: 4; 1 bowl per serving

Ingredients

- 1 cup rolled oats, old-fashioned
- 2 tablespoons chopped dried cherries
- ½ teaspoon salt
- 4 teaspoons coconut sugar

- 1 cup water

- 2 tablespoons toasted chopped walnuts
- 1 teaspoon lemon zest
- 4 tablespoons reduced-fat cream cheese

Directions

- Take a large bowl, place oats in it, add salt, pour in the water, and then stir until combined.
- Cover the bowl with its lid, place it in the refrigerator and then let the oats rest for a minimum of 8 hours or overnight.
- When ready to eat, bring oats to room temperature, stir until just mixed, and then divide evenly among four bowls.
- Sprinkle with sugar, top with cheese, walnuts, and cream cheese, sprinkle with lemon zest and then serve.

Blackberry and Ginger Overnight Bulgur

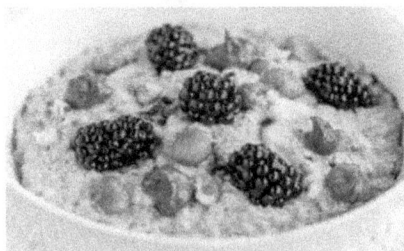

Nutritional Information per Serving

Calories: 110 calories
Fat: 1g
Sat. Fat: 0.5g
Carbohydrates: 22.5g
Protein: 4g
Fiber: 1.5g

Prep Time: 8 hours and 10 minutes | Cook Time: 0 minutes | Servings: 4; 1 bowl per serving

Ingredients

- 1 cup bulgur
- 8 tablespoons honey, organic
- 1 cup blackberries, fresh

- 1 teaspoon ground ginger
- 1 1/3 cup coconut yogurt, low-fat
- 12 tablespoons coconut milk, unsweetened, low-fat

Directions

- Take a large bowl, place bulgur in it, add honey and ginger, and then pour in the milk and yogurt.
- Stir until well combined, cover the bowl with its lid, place it in the refrigerator and then let the bulgur rest for a minimum of 8 hours or overnight.
- When ready to eat, bring bulgur to room temperature, stir until just mixed, and then divide evenly among four bowls.
- Top the bulgur with the blackberries and then serve.

Quinoa and Chia Oatmeal Mix

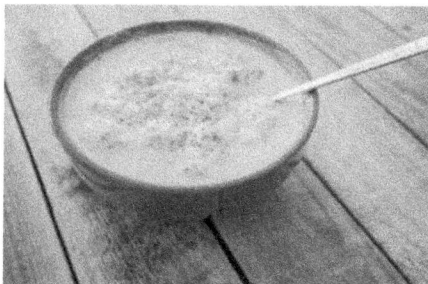

Nutritional Information per Serving

Calories: 172 calories
Fat: 3.2g
Sat. Fat: 0.5g
Carbohydrates: 28g
Protein: 5.2g
Fiber: 4.1g

Prep Time: 10 minutes | Cook Time: 15 minutes | Servings: 4; 1 bowl per serving

Ingredients

For the Oatmeal Mix:

- 1 cup rolled oats, old fashioned
- ½ cup dried fruit mixture
- ½ cup rolled wheat
- ¼ cup chia seeds

- ½ teaspoon ground cinnamon

For Each Serving:

- ½ tablespoon chopped walnuts
- 1 tablespoon honey, raw

- ½ cup quinoa
- ¼ teaspoon salt

- ½ tablespoon sliced almonds
- 1 cup almond milk, unsweetened, low-fat

Directions

- Prepare the mix and for this, take a large bowl, place oats in it, and then add dried fruit mix, wheat, chia seeds, and quinoa.
- Add salt and cinnamon, stir until well mixed, and then store it by transferring the mixture into an air-tight container.
- When ready to eat, take a small saucepan, place it over medium heat, add ¼ cup of the oatmeal mix and 1 cup milk and then bring the mixture to a boil.
- Then switch heat to low level and simmer the oatmeal for 10 to 15 minutes until thickened to the desired level, covering the pan partially.
- When done, remove the pan from heat, cover the pan with a lid and let the mixture stand for 5 minutes.
- Transfer the oatmeal mixture into a bowl, drizzle with honey, sprinkle walnuts and almonds on top, and then serve.

Quinoa with Blueberry and Lemon

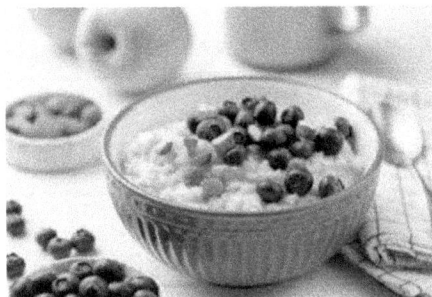

Nutritional Information per Serving

Calories: 269 calories
Fat: 3.6g
Sat. Fat: 0.4g
Carbohydrates: 49.3g
Protein: 11.7g
Fiber: 4.4g

Prep Time: 10 minutes | Cook Time: 20 minutes | Servings: 4; 1 bowl per serving

Ingredients

- 1 cup blueberries, fresh
- ½ of a lemon, zested
- 1 cups quinoa, rinsed

- ½ tablespoon and ½ teaspoon flax seeds
- 3 tablespoons honey, raw
- 2 cups almond milk, unsweetened,

- 1/8 teaspoon salt   low-fat

Directions

- Take a medium saucepan, place it over medium heat, pour in the milk, and then cook for 3 minutes until thoroughly warmed.
- Add quinoa, stir in salt, switch heat to medium-low level and then cook for 20 minutes until the quinoa has absorbed all the milk.
- Then remove the pan from heat, stir in lemon zest and honey and then fold in berries until just mixed.
- Divide the quinoa evenly among four bowls and then serve.

Yogurt with Blueberries and Honey

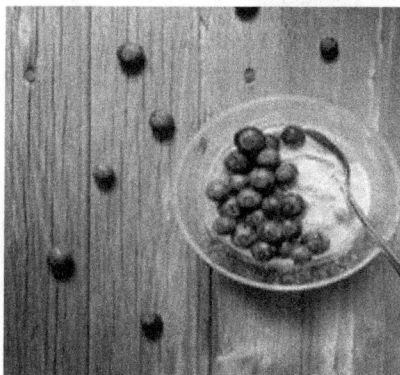

Nutritional Information per Serving

Calories: 196 calories
Fat: 1.1g
Sat. Fat: 0.3g
Carbohydrates: 24.6g
Protein: 23.5g
Fiber: 1.8g

Fat: 100 g

Prep Time: 10 minutes | Cook Time: 10 minutes | Servings: 4; 1 bowl per serving
Ingredients

- 2 cups blueberries, fresh
- 4 teaspoons honey
- 4 cups coconut yogurt or Greek yogurt, low-fat

Directions

- Take a small bowl, place 1 cup yogurt in it, top with ½ cup berries and then drizzle with 1 teaspoon honey.
- Assemble three more bowls in the same manner and then serve.

Chapter 7
Lunch

Tuna Patties

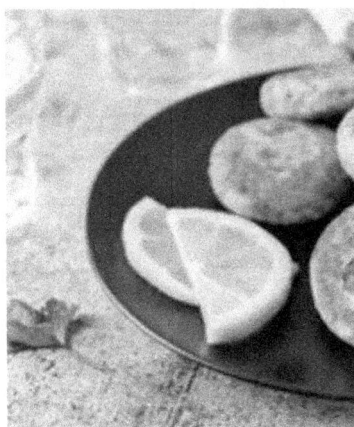

Nutritional Information per Serving

Calories: 216 calories
Fat: 12g
Sat. Fat: 3g
Carbohydrates: 32g
Protein: 12g
Fiber: 2g

Prep Time: 10 minutes | Cook Time: 15 minutes | Servings: 4; 2 patties per serving

Ingredients

- 14 ounces canned tuna, water-packed, drained
- 2 shallots, peeled, chopped
- 6 tablespoons bread crumbs
- 2 tablespoons parsley, chopped
- 4 tablespoons chives, chopped
- 2 tablespoons scallions, chopped
- ½ teaspoon ground black pepper
- 2 tablespoons scallions, chopped
- ½ teaspoon ground black pepper
- 8 tablespoons whole-wheat flour
- 2/3 teaspoon salt
- 4 tablespoons grated parmesan cheese
- 2 medium eggs, at room temperature
- 2 tablespoons sour cream

- 2 tablespoons olive oil

Directions

- Take a medium bowl, place tuna in it, add chopped shallots, bread crumbs, parsley, chives, scallion, black pepper, 4 tablespoons flour, salt, cheese, egg, and sour cream.
- Stir until well combined, shape the mixture into 8 evenly sized patties and then dredge in the remaining flour.
- Take a medium skillet pan, add oil and when hot, add prepared patties and then cook for 5 to 7 minutes per side until golden brown.
- Serve the tuna patties with a green salad.

Mediterranean Salmon

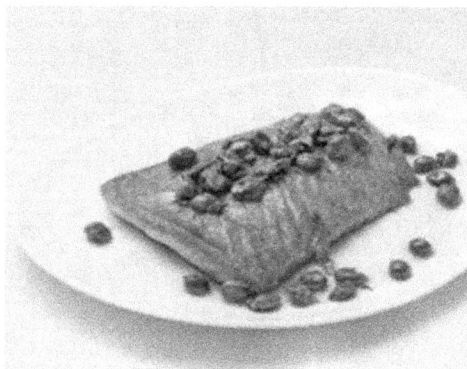

Nutritional Information per Serving

Calories: 301 calories
Fat: 15g
Sat. Fat: 2g
Carbohydrates: 5g
Protein: 35g
Fiber: 2g

Prep Time: 10 minutes | Cook Time: 25 minutes | Servings: 4; 1 piece per serving

Ingredients

- 1 ½ pound salmon fillet
- 1 tablespoon chopped dill
- ¼ teaspoon salt
- 2 teaspoons minced garlic

- 1 tablespoon capers
- 2 tablespoons lemon juice
- 1 tablespoon olive oil

- 1/3 cup whole-grain mustard
- 1 lemon, sliced

Directions

- Switch on the oven, then set it to 400 degrees F and let it preheat.
- Meanwhile, take a baking sheet and then place salmon fillet skin-side-down on it.
- Take a small bowl, place garlic, capers, dill, salt, and mustard in it, pour in the lemon juice and oil, and then stir until mixed.
- Brush the garlic mixture generously on the salmon, top with lemon slices, and then bake for 20 to 25 minutes until tender.
- Cut the salmon into four pieces and then serve.

Shrimp Linguine

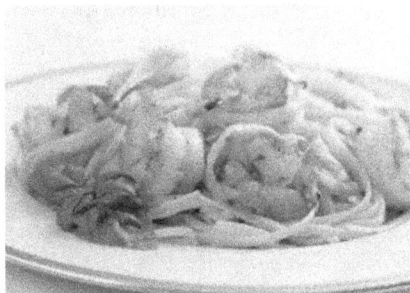

Nutritional Information per Serving

Calories: 231 calories
Fat: 8g
Sat. Fat: 1.5g
Carbohydrates: 24g
Protein: 1.5g
Fiber: 14g

Prep Time: 10 minutes | Cook Time: 25 minutes | Servings: 4; 1 plate per serving

Ingredients

- 12 ounces whole-wheat linguine
- 1 ½ pound medium shrimp, peeled, deveined
- ½ of a large white onion, peeled, chopped
- 1/3 cup minced parsley
- ½ teaspoon crushed red pepper flakes
- ½ teaspoon salt
- 2 tablespoons lemon juice
- ¼ teaspoon dried oregano

- 1 teaspoon minced garlic
- 2/3 cup chopped roasted sweet red peppers
- 2-1/4 ounces sliced olives

- ½ teaspoon ground black pepper
- 5 tablespoons olive oil
- 8 tablespoons crumbled feta cheese
- 1/3 cup chicken broth

Directions

- Prepare the pasta, and for this, take a large pot half full with water, place it over medium-high heat and then bring it to a boil.
- Add the pasta, cook it for 8 to 10 minutes until tender, then drain it well and reserve ½ cup of a cooking liquid, set aside until required.
- While pasta cooks, take a large skillet pan, place it over medium heat, add oil and when hot, add onion and cook for 2 to 3 minutes until onions begin to soften.
- Add shrimps, stir until just mixed, cook for 3 to 4 minutes per side until pink, stir in garlic and continue cooking for 1 minute.
- Switch heat to medium-low level, add olives, sweet red peppers, salt, parsley, black pepper, and oregano, pour in the reserved cooking liquid and stir until mixed.
- Add the cooked pasta along with cheese, drizzle with the lemon juice, stir until well mixed, cook for 3 to 4 minutes until the cheese has melted, and then serve.

Vegetarian Pasta Carbonara

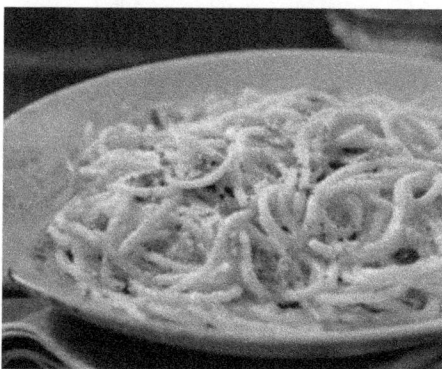

Nutritional Information per Serving

Calories: 300 calories
Fat: 11.5g
Sat. Fat: 3.5g
Carbohydrates: 36.5g
Protein: 12.5g
Fiber: 2.5g

Prep Time: 10 minutes | Cook Time: 22 minutes | Servings: 4; 1 bowl per serving

Ingredients

- 6 ounces whole-wheat spaghetti
- 1 tablespoon pine nuts, toasted
- 8 cherry tomatoes, halved
- 2 small zucchinis, cut into 1/3-inch-thick sticks
- ¼ teaspoon salt
- 1 teaspoon minced garlic
- 1/8 teaspoon ground black pepper
- 2 egg yolks, at room temperature
- 1 tablespoon olive oil and more as needed
- ½ cup grated parmesan, low-fat
- 3 tablespoons pasta water

Directions

- Take a large pot half full with salted water, place it over medium-high heat and then bring it to a boil.
- Add pasta, cook it for 10 to 12 minutes until tender, and then drain it into a colander, reserving 3 tablespoons of the pasta water.
- While pasta cooks, take a large frying pan, place it over medium heat, add oil and when hot, add zucchini and then cook for 5 to 8 minutes until nicely browned.
- Stir in garlic, cook for 1 minute, add tomatoes, stir in 1/8 teaspoon salt and then remove the pan from heat.
- Prepare the sauce and for this, take a medium bowl, place egg yolks in it, add cheese, black pepper, and remaining salt, whisk until smooth, and then whisk in the reserved pasta water until creamy sauce comes together.
- When zucchini has cooked, add the drained pasta, toss until combined, and then cook for 1 minute until thoroughly warmed.
- Pour in the prepared sauce, toss until mixed, sprinkle pine nuts and some more black pepper on top.
- Divide the pasta carbonara evenly among four plates and then serve.

Bean Burgers

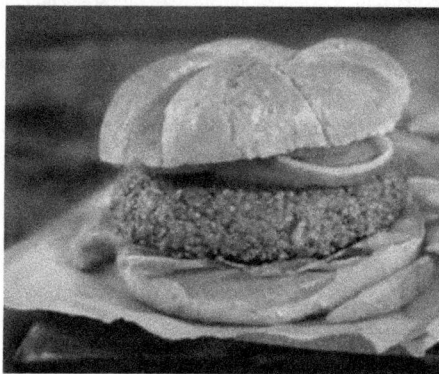

Nutritional Information per Serving

Calories: 323.3 calories
Fat: 23.3g
Sat. Fat: 4.4g
Carbohydrates: 16.6g
Protein: 11.1g
Fiber: 4g

Prep Time: 10 minutes | Cook Time: 15 minutes | Servings: 4 burgers; 1 burger per serving

Ingredients

For the Bean Patties:

- 24 ounces canned pink beans, rinsed
- ½ of a medium white onion, minced
- ½ cup chickpea flour
- 1/3 teaspoon ground black pepper
- 1 teaspoon minced garlic
- 1/3 teaspoon dried sage
- ¾ teaspoon salt
- ¾ teaspoon dried oregano
- ¾ cup chopped parsley
- ¼ cup olive oil
- 2 medium eggs, at room temperature
- For the Burgers:
- 4 whole-wheat burger buns, halved, toasted
- 4 leaves of lettuce
- 4 slices of tomato
- 1 medium avocado, peeled, pitted, diced

Directions

- Prepare the bean patties, and for this, take a large bowl, place beans and onion in it and then add chickpea flour, black pepper, garlic, sage, salt, oregano, parsley, and eggs.

- Stir until well combined, and then shape the mixture into four evenly sized patties.
- Take a medium skillet pan, place it over medium-high heat, pour in the oil, and when hot, add the prepared bean patties and then cook for 6 to 8 minutes per side until golden brown.
- Assemble the burgers and for this, cut each burger bun in half and then toast the slices.
- Layer the bottom half of a burger bun with a lettuce leaf, and then place a bean patty on it.
- Top the bean patty with a tomato slice and avocado, drizzle with favorite sauce from the 'Sauces, Dips, and Dressing' section, and then cover with the top half of the bun.
- Assemble the remaining burgers in the same manner and then serve.

Herby Black Bean Salad with Feta Cheese

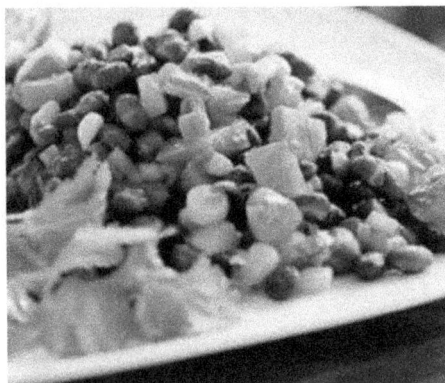

Nutritional Information per Serving

Calories: 245 calories
Fat: 15g
Sat. Fat: 3g
Carbohydrates: 23g
Protein: 9g
Fiber: 8g

Prep Time: 10 minutes | Cook Time: 0 minutes | Servings: 4; 1 bowl per serving

Ingredients

- 1 cup canned black beans, rinsed
- 2 roasted green peppers, chopped
- 2 cups arugula
- 2 cups diced tomatoes
- ¼ cup basil leaves
- 2 tablespoons pickled jalapenos
- ¼ teaspoon ground black pepper

- 2 scallions, chopped
- ¼ cup olives pitted
- ½ cup parsley leaves
- ½ teaspoon minced garlic
- ¼ teaspoon salt

- 4 tablespoons crumbled feta cheese, low-fat
- 2 tablespoons olive oil
- 2 tablespoons sesame seeds, toasted

Directions

- Take a medium bowl, place black beans and roasted green peppers along with arugula, scallion, olives, and tomatoes.
- Add remaining ingredients, toss until well combined, then divide the salad evenly among four bowls and serve.

Tomato, Basil, and Chickpea Salad

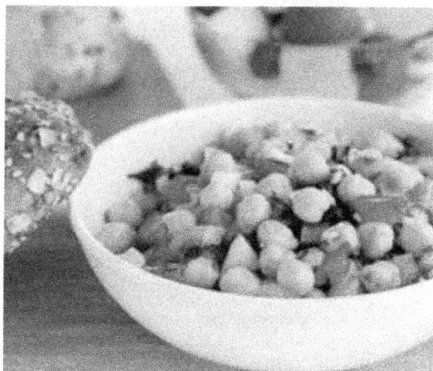

Nutritional Information per Serving

Calories: 354 calories
Fat: 18g
Sat. Fat: 3g
Carbohydrates: 35g
Protein: 13g
Fiber: 7g

Prep Time: 10 minutes | Cook Time: 10 minutes | Servings: 4; 1 bowl per serving

Ingredients

- 16 ounces canned chickpeas, drained, rinsed
- 3 small white onions, peeled, sliced
- 6 green onions, sliced

- 2 cups chopped cilantro
- 3 large tomatoes, chopped
- 1 cup basil leaves, chopped
- 4 tablespoons olive oil

- 3 small red pepper, chopped
- 1 teaspoon salt
- 4 tablespoons sesame seeds
- 4 teaspoons balsamic vinegar

Directions

- Take a large bowl, place chickpeas in it, and then add white onion, green onions, red pepper, and tomatoes.
- Season with salt, add cilantro and basil, drizzle with balsamic vinegar and then toss until just mixed.
- Sprinkle sesame seeds over the salad and then serve.

Tabouli Salad

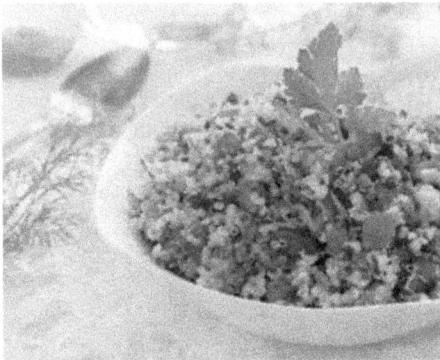

Nutritional Information per Serving

Calories: 257 calories
Fat: 13.3g
Sat. Fat: 4g
Carbohydrates: 34g
Protein: 4.3g
Fiber: 4.1g

Prep Time: 40 minutes | Cook Time: 0 minutes | Servings: 4; 1 bowl per serving

Ingredients

- ½ cup bulgur wheat
- 1 large cucumber, chopped
- 4 medium tomatoes, chopped
- 2 bunches of parsley, destemmed, chopped
- 4 tablespoons lemon juice
- 4 green onions, green and white part separated, chopped
- 1 cup mint leaves, chopped
- ½ teaspoon salt
- 3 tablespoons olive oil

Directions

- Wash the bulgur wheat, place it in a medium bowl, cover with water and then let the wheat soak for 5 to 7 minutes.
- Meanwhile, chop the tomatoes, place them into a colander and let them rest until excess juice has drained completely.
- Then take a large bowl, place tomatoes in it, and then add cucumber, green onion, parsley, and mint leaves.
- Add bulgur, season with salt, drizzle with lemon juice and olive oil, toss just mixed, and then cover the bowl with its lid.
- Place the bowl in the refrigerator, let it rest for 30 minutes, and then divide it evenly among four bowls.
- Serve the salad with Baba Ghanoush or hummus which you can prepare from the 'Sauces, Dips, and Dressing' section.

Roasted Eggplants

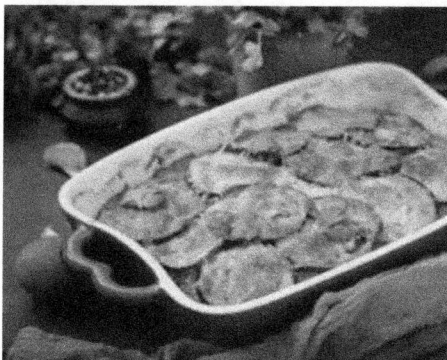

Nutritional Information per Serving

Calories: 249.7 calories
Fat: 17.2g
Sat. Fat: 4g
Carbohydrates: 18.7g
Protein: 5g
Fiber: 9g

Prep Time: 15 minutes | Cook Time: 1 hour and 10 minutes | Servings: 4

Ingredients

- 2 large eggplants, about 2-pounds total
- 4 medium tomatoes, chopped
- ½ teaspoon ground black pepper
- ¼ cup chopped mint
- ¼ cup olive oil

- 5 cloves of garlic, peeled, minced
- 1 teaspoon salt
- ¼ cup chopped parsley
- 3 tablespoons apple cider vinegar
- 4 tablespoons crumbled feta cheese, low-fat

Directions

- Cut the eggplant into ½-inch thick slices, place them in a large bowl, season with ½ teaspoon salt and then toss until just mixed.
- Take a large skillet pan, place it over medium-high heat, add 2 tablespoons of oil and when hot, spread eggplant slices in a single layer and then cook for 3 minutes per side until golden brown.
- Transfer the browned eggplant slices to a plate lined with a paper towel and then repeat with the remaining eggplant slices.
- Meanwhile, switch on the oven, set it to 350 degrees F, and let it preheat.
- When eggplant slices have cooked, return the skillet pan over medium heat, add garlic and cook for 1 to 2 minutes until fragrant and softened.
- Add tomatoes, season with black pepper and remaining salt, add vinegar and honey and then cook for 15 minutes or until thicken sauce comes together.
- Remove the pan from the heat, take a medium baking dish, spread a few tablespoons of the sauce in its bottom, and then drizzle with a little oil.
- Layer with eggplant slices in a single layer and sprinkle with some parsley, mint, and feta cheese.
- Spread some of the prepared tomato sauce over the eggplant layer and then continue layering remaining eggplant slices with parsley, mint, feta cheese, and tomato sauce until all of these ingredients have used up.
- Use a spatula to press down the eggplant slices, drizzle vinegar on top and then bake for 45 minutes until done.
- Sprinkle some more feta cheese on top and then serve.

Mediterranean Cauliflower Pizza

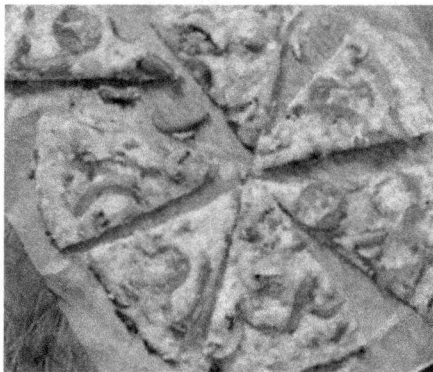

Nutritional Information per Serving

Calories: 200 calories
Fat: 14g
Sat. Fat: 4.7g
Carbohydrates: 10.2g
Protein: 10.8g
Fiber: 3.2g

Prep Time: 15 minutes | Cook Time: 35 minutes | Servings: 1 pizza; 1 slice per serving

Ingredients

- 2 pounds head of cauliflower, chopped into florets
- 6 sun-dried tomatoes, oil-packed, drained, chopped
- ½ teaspoon dried oregano
- ⅓ cup olives, pitted, sliced
- ½ teaspoon ground black pepper
- ¼ teaspoon salt
- 1 tablespoon and 1 teaspoon olive oil, divided
- 1 large lemon
- 1 large egg, at room temperature, beaten
- ¼ cup sliced basil
- 1 cup shredded mozzarella cheese, low-fat

Directions

- Switch on the oven, then set it to 450 degrees F and let it preheat.
- Meanwhile, take a pizza pan, line it with parchment paper, and set it aside until required.
- Plug in a food processor, place cauliflower florets in it, and then pulse until mixture resembles rice.
- Take a large skillet pan, place it over medium heat, add 1 tablespoon oil and when hot, add cauliflower mixture, stir in salt and then cook for 8 to 10 minutes until golden brown.

- Then transfer the cauliflower mixture into a large bowl and then let it cool at room temperature for 10 minutes.
- Meanwhile, peel the lemon, remove and discard its white pith, remove the seeds, and then cut the lemon into segments.
- Drain the juice from the lemon segment, place the lemon pieces into a bowl, add olives and tomatoes and then toss until combined.
- When the cauliflower mixture has cooled, add cheese, oregano, and egg, stir until well combined, spoon the mixture into the prepared pizza pan, and then spread it evenly.
- Drizzle the remaining oil on top, place it into the oven, and then bake for 10 to 15 minutes until the crust begins to turn brown.
- Then scatter the prepared olives-tomato-lemon mixture over the top of the baked crust, season with the black pepper, and continue baking the pizza for 8 to 14 minutes until done.
- Scatter basil leaves on top, cut into slices and then serve.

Quinoa and Avocado Salad

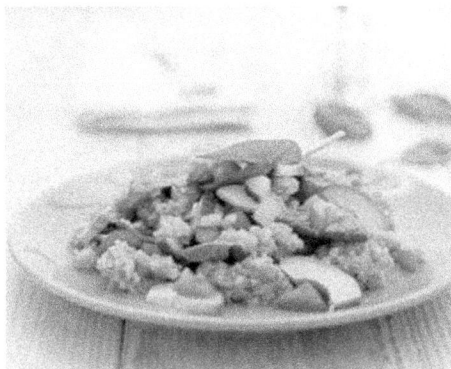

Nutritional Information per Serving

Calories: 236 calories
Fat: 5.7g
Sat. Fat: 1.8g
Carbohydrates: 25.2g
Protein: 5.2g
Fiber: 6.7g

Prep Time: 25 minutes | Cook Time: 15 minutes | Servings: 4; 1 bowl per serving

Ingredients

For the Salad Dressing:

For the Salad:

- ¾ teaspoon salt
- ¾ teaspoon garlic powder

- 1 medium avocado, peeled, pitted, chopped

- ¼ teaspoon ground black pepper
- 2 tablespoons avocado oil
- 3 tablespoons lime juice

- ¾ cup quinoa, uncooked, rinsed
- ½ cup grape tomatoes, halved
- ½ cup spinach leaves, fresh
- 1 scallion, sliced
- ¾ cup diced cucumber
- ¼ cup chopped cilantro
- 1 ½ cup water

Directions

- Prepare the quinoa, and for this, take a medium pot, pour water in it, place it over medium-high heat and bring it to a boil.
- Then switch heat to medium level, add quinoa and then cook for 8 to 15 minutes until all the liquid has been absorbed by the quinoa.
- Meanwhile, prepare the salad dressing and for this, take a small bowl, place all the ingredients for the dressing in it and then stir until combined, set aside until required.
- Remove the pot from heat, cover it with its lid, let the quinoa rest for 5 minutes, and then fluff it with a fork.
- Stir ¼ teaspoon salt into the quinoa, and then let the quinoa rest for 15 minutes at room temperature.
- Take a large bowl, place quinoa in it, add the remaining ingredients of the salad in it, drizzle with the prepared salad dressing, and then stir gently until just mixed.
- Divide the salad between 4 bowls and then serve.

Chickpea and Quinoa Bowl

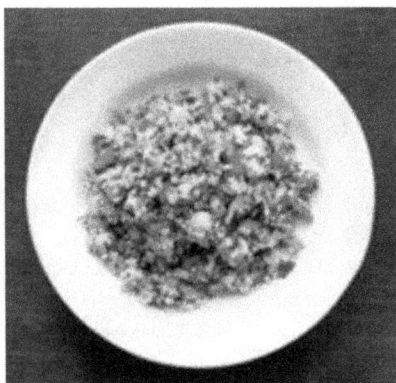

Nutritional Information per Serving

Calories: 273 calories
Fat: 24.3g
Sat. Fat: 4.3g
Carbohydrates: 49g
Protein: 12.7g
Fiber: 7.7g

Prep Time: 25 minutes | Cook Time: 15 minutes | Servings: 4; 1 bowl per serving

Ingredients

For the Salad Dressing:

- 7 ounces roasted red peppers, rinsed
- ¼ cup slivered almonds
- 2 tablespoons olive oil
- ¼ teaspoon crushed red pepper
- ½ teaspoon ground cumin
- ½ teaspoon minced garlic

For the Salad:

- ½ cup quinoa, uncooked, rinsed
- ¼ cup Kalamata olives, chopped
- 12 ounces canned chickpeas, drained, rinsed
- ¼ cup chopped red onion
- ½ cup diced cucumber
- ½ teaspoon paprika
- 1 ½ tablespoon olive oil
- ¼ cup crumbled feta cheese, low-fat
- 2 tablespoons chopped parsley
- 1 cup water

Directions

- Prepare the quinoa, and for this, take a medium pot, pour water in it, place it over medium-high heat and bring it to a boil.
- Then switch heat to medium level, add quinoa and then cook for 8 to 15 minutes until all the liquid has been absorbed by the quinoa.

- Meanwhile, prepare the salad dressing and for this, plug in a food processor, add all the ingredients for the salad dressing in it and then pulse until smooth.
- Remove the pot from heat, cover it with its lid, let the quinoa rest for 5 minutes, and then fluff it with a fork.
- Stir ¼ teaspoon salt into the quinoa, and then let the quinoa rest for 15 minutes at room temperature.
- Take a large bowl, place quinoa in it, add the remaining ingredients of the salad in it, drizzle with the prepared salad dressing, and then stir gently until just mixed.
- Divide the salad between 4 bowls and then serve.

Chapter 8

Snacks

Pineapple and Green Smoothie

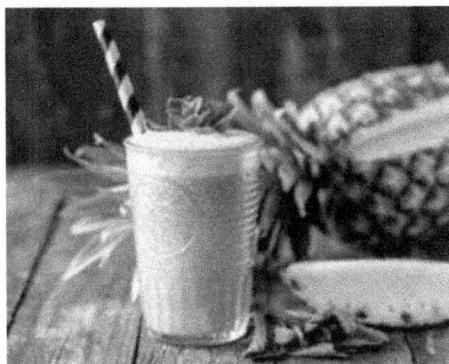

**Nutritional
Information per
Serving**

Calories: 195 calories
Fat: 3g
Sat. Fat: 1.1g
Carbohydrates: 32.6g
Protein: 9.3g
Fiber: 5.1g

Prep Time: 5 minutes | Cook Time: 0 minutes | Servings: 1 glass

Ingredients

- ¼ cup almond milk, unsweetened
- ¼ cup Greek yogurt, low-fat
- ½ cup baby spinach, fresh
- ¼ cup pineapple chunks, frozen
- 1 frozen banana, peeled
- 1 Medjool date, pitted
- 1 teaspoon chia seeds

Directions

- Plugin the food processor and then pour milk and yogurt in its jar.
- Add spinach, pineapple, banana, honey, and chia seeds, and then pulse for 30 seconds or more until smooth.
- Pour the smoothie into a glass and then serve.

Tahini and Date Shake

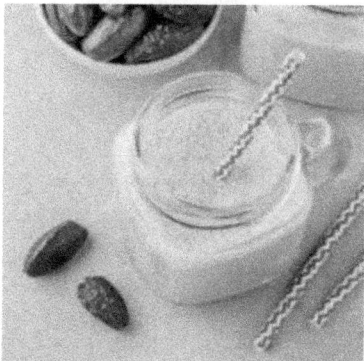

Nutritional Information per Serving

Calories: 199.4 calories
Fat: 8.2g
Sat. Fat: 1.6g
Carbohydrates: 27.7g
Protein: 3.7g
Fiber: 5.6g

Prep Time: 5 minutes | Cook Time: 0 minutes | Servings: 1

Ingredients

- ¼ cup ice cubes
- ½ cup almond milk, unsweetened
- 1 frozen banana, peeled
- 1 ½ tablespoon tahini
- 1 Medjool date, pitted
- ¼ teaspoon ground cinnamon

Directions

- Plugin the food processor, add ice cubes, and then pour in the milk.
- Add banana, tahini, date, and cinnamon, and then pulse for 30 seconds or more until smooth.
- Pour the smoothie into a glass and then serve.

Chia and Pomegranate Smoothie

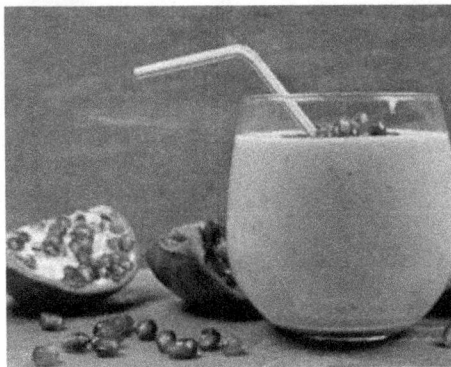

Nutritional Information per Serving

Calories: 208 calories
Fat: 4.6g
Sat. Fat: 1.3g
Carbohydrates: 32.7g
Protein: 8.8g
Fiber: 4.9g

Prep Time: 5 minutes | Cook Time: 0 minutes | Servings: 1

Ingredients

- ½ cup pomegranate juice, chilled
- ¼ cup Greek yogurt, low-fat
- ½ of a frozen banana, peeled
- 1 tablespoon chia seeds

Directions

- Plugin the food processor and then pour in the juice and yogurt.
- Add banana and chia seeds, and then pulse for 30 seconds or more until smooth.
- Pour the smoothie into a glass and then serve.

Orange Salad

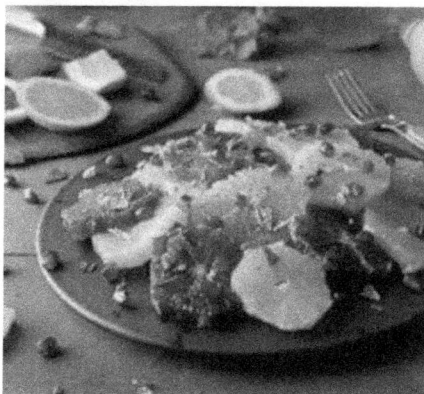

Nutritional Information per Serving

Calories: 186 calories
Fat: 11.7g
Sat. Fat: 1.6g
Carbohydrates: 21.4g
Protein: 1.8g
Fiber: 4.5g

Prep Time: 5 minutes | Cook Time: 0 minutes | Servings: 4; 1 plate per serving

Ingredients

- 4 oranges
- 1 small white onion, peeled, diced
- 3 blood oranges
- 1/8 teaspoon salt

- 2 tablespoons lemon juice
- 1/8 teaspoon ground black pepper
- 10 dried black olives
- 3 tablespoons olive oil

Directions

- Prepare the oranges and for this, cut off a small piece from its top and bottom, remove the skin and white pith, and then cut the oranges into horizontal slices.
- Take a small bowl, place onion slices in it, add salt, lemon juice, and olive oil and then stir until combined.
- Spoon the onion mixture over the orange slices, season with black pepper, and then scatter olives from the top.
- Serve straight away.

Mediterranean Fruit Salad

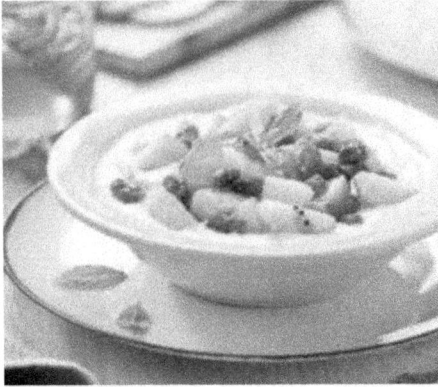

Nutritional Information per Serving

Calories: 201 calories
Fat: 0.9g
Sat. Fat: 0.1g
Carbohydrates: 51.3g
Protein: 2.6g
Fiber: 9.1g

Prep Time: 5 minutes | Cook Time: 0 minutes | Servings: 4; 1 bowl per serving

Ingredients

- 2 medium pears, cored, chopped
- 24 grapes, seedless
- 2 medium apples, cored, chopped
- 4 kiwi fruits, chopped
- 2 medium peaches, chopped
- 2 oranges, peeled, deseeded, chopped
- 1 cup Greek yogurt, low-fat

Directions

- Take a large bowl and then place pears, grapes, apples, kiwi, peaches, and oranges.
- Add yogurt, stir until well mixed and then divide the salad evenly among four bowls.
- Serve straight away.

Trail Mix

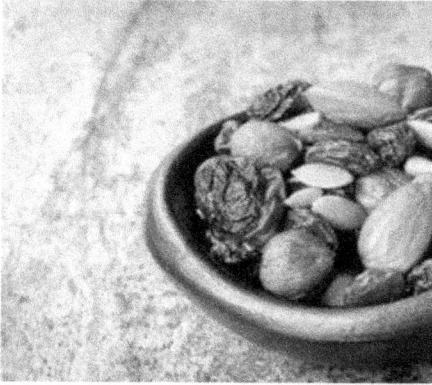

Nutritional Information per Serving

Calories: 218.5 calories
Fat: 12.4g
Sat. Fat: 2.3g
Carbohydrates: 21.3g
Protein: 5.5g
Fiber: 5.5g

Prep Time: 10 minutes | Cook Time: 0 minutes | Servings: 4; 1 bowl per serving

Ingredients

For the Trail Mix:

- 2 tablespoons sunflower seeds, unsalted
- ½ cup almonds
- 3 tablespoons chocolate chips, semi-sweetened
- 2 tablespoons whole dried cherries
- 12 apricots, dried

For Each Serving:

- ½ cup almond milk, unsweetened, low-fat

Directions

- Take a large bowl, place sunflower seeds, almonds, chocolate chips, cherries, and apricot, and then stir until mixed.
- Transfer the prepared trail mix into a resealable glass container and then store it at room temperature until required.
- When ready to serve, transfer ½ cup of the trail mix into a bowl, pour in ½ cup milk, and then serve.

Flatbread Crackers

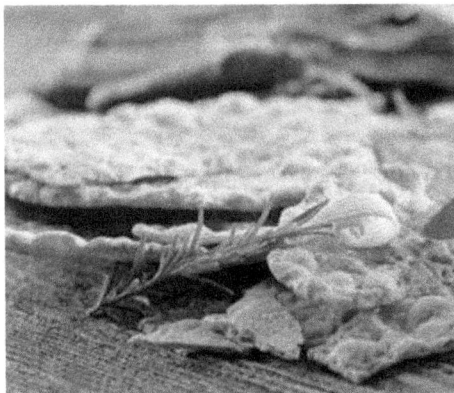

Nutritional Information per Serving

Calories: 190 calories
Fat: 6g
Sat. Fat: 1g
Carbohydrates: 29g
Protein: 4g
Fiber: 1.2g

Prep Time: 10 minutes | Cook Time: 10 minutes | Servings: 4

Ingredients

- 1 ½ cups whole-wheat flour
- 1 teaspoon ground black pepper
- 2 teaspoons dried thyme
- 1 teaspoon coconut sugar

- 1 teaspoon salt
- 2 tablespoons olive oil
- ½ cup water, chilled

Directions

- Switch on the oven, then set it to 450 degrees F and let it preheat.
- Meanwhile, plug in a food processor, add flour in it, add salt, sugar, black pepper, and thyme, and then pour in olive oil.
- Pulse until well mixed, and then slowly blend in water for 10 seconds until a sticky dough comes together.
- Transfer the dough to a clean working space dusted with flour, shape it into a ball, divide the ball into four evenly sized portions, and then let the dough portions rest for 10 minutes.
- Meanwhile, take a baking sheet, line it with a parchment sheet, and set it aside until required.

- Working on one portion of dough at a time, roll it as thin as possible, transfer it to the prepared baking sheet and bake for 4 to 5 minutes per side until golden brown.
- When done, switch off the oven and then let the cracker rest in the oven for 1 to 2 hours until dried and crisp.
- Then break the crispy cracker into pieces and repeat with the remaining flour portions.
- Serve the crackers with your favorite dip, which you can prepare from the 'Sauces, Dips, and Dressing' section.

Roasted Chickpeas

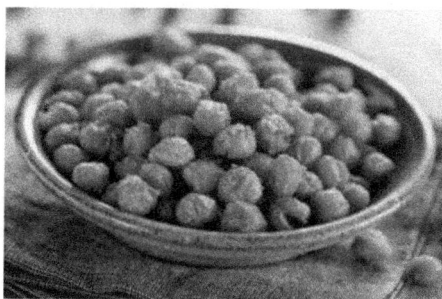

Nutritional Information per Serving

Calories: 208 calories
Fat: 9.4g
Sat. Fat: 1.1g
Carbohydrates: 23.8g
Protein: 6.7g
Fiber: 6.8g

Prep Time: 10 minutes | Cook Time: 30 minutes | Servings: 4

Ingredients

- 15 ounces canned chickpeas, drained, rinsed
- ¼ teaspoon garlic powder
- ½ teaspoon salt
- 2 tablespoons olive oil
- 1 teaspoon dried oregano
- 2 teaspoons red wine vinegar
- ¼ teaspoon ground black pepper
- 2 teaspoons lemon juice

Directions

- Switch on the oven, then set it to 425 degrees F and let it preheat.
- Meanwhile, take a large baking sheet and then line it with the parchment.

- Spread the chickpeas into the prepared baking sheet in a single layer and then roast for 20 minutes until golden brown, stirring halfway.
- Meanwhile, prepare the dressing and for this, take a large bowl, place garlic powder, salt, black pepper, and oregano in it, pour in lemon juice and olive oil, and then whisk until well combined.
- When the chickpeas have roasted, transfer them into the bowl containing prepared dressing and then toss until coated.
- Spoon the chickpeas into the baking sheet, spread them in a single layer, and then roast them for 10 minutes, stirring halfway.
- Let the roasted chickpeas cool for 5 minutes and then serve.

Baked Zucchini Sticks

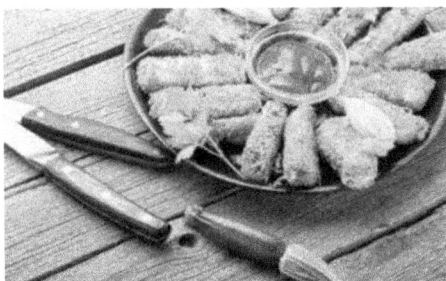

Nutritional Information per Serving

Calories: 132 calories
Fat: 6.6g
Sat. Fat: 3.6g
Carbohydrates: 9.6g
Protein: 10.8g
Fiber: 3.2g

Prep Time: 10 minutes | Cook Time: 25 minutes | Servings: 4

Ingredients

- 4 large zucchinis, ends trimmed, cut into lengthwise sticks
- 6 tablespoons olive oil

For the Topping:

- ¾ teaspoon salt

- 3 teaspoons dried thyme
- 1 teaspoon paprika
- 2 teaspoons dried oregano
- 1 teaspoon ground black pepper
- 1 cup grated parmesan cheese, low-fat

Directions

- Switch on the oven, then set it to 350 degrees F and let it preheat.

- Meanwhile, take a shallow dish, place all the ingredients for the topping in it and then stir until just mixed.
- Take a large baking sheet, place a wire rack on it, and then brush it with oil.
- Arrange the prepared zucchini sticks skin-side-down on the wire rack in a single layer, brush them with oil and then sprinkle with the prepared topping mixture until coated.
- Place the prepared baking tray into the oven to bake for 20 minutes until golden crisp, then switch on the broiler and continue baking the zucchini sticks for 3 minutes.
- When done, serve the zucchini sticks with your favorite sauce, which you can prepare from the 'Sauces, Dips, and Dressing' section.

Fish Sticks

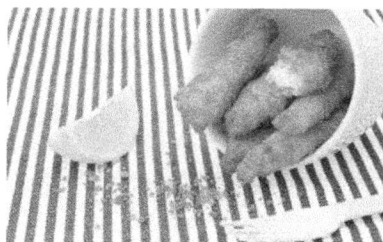

Nutritional Information per Serving

Calories: 238 calories
Fat: 7.6g
Sat. Fat: 2.2g
Carbohydrates: 16g
Protein: 27.2g
Fiber: 1.2g

Prep Time: 15 minutes | Cook Time: 18 minutes | Servings: 16 fish sticks; 4 fish sticks per serving

Ingredients

- ½ cup whole-wheat breadcrumbs
- 1½ pounds cod, skinless
- ½ cup whole-wheat flour
- 1 teaspoon salt
- 1 teaspoon dried oregano
- 1 teaspoon ground black pepper
- 1 teaspoon sweet paprika

- 1 lemon, zested
- 1 large egg, at room temperature
- ½ cup grated Parmesan cheese, low-fat
- ½ of a lemon, juiced
- 4 tablespoons olive oil
- 1 tablespoon chopped parsley

Directions

- Switch on the oven, then set it to 450 degrees F and let it preheat.
- Rinse the fish, pat dry with paper towels, season well with salt, and then cut it into 3-inch-long slices, each about 1 ½ inch thick.
- Take a small bowl, place paprika, oregano, and black pepper in it, stir until well mixed and then sprinkle this mixture on the fish sticks until coated.
- Take a shallow dish and then place flour in it.
- Take another shallow dish, crack the egg in it and then whisk until blended.
- Take another shallow dish, place breadcrumbs in it, add lemon zest and parmesan cheese, and then stir until mixed.
- Working on one fish stick at a time, dredge it in flour, dip into the blended eggs and then dredge in the breadcrumb's mixture until well coated.
- Take a large baking sheet, grease it with oil, arrange the prepared fish sticks on it, brush some more oil on top of the prepared fish sticks and then bake for 15 minutes until golden brown, turning halfway.
- Then switch on the broiler and continue baking the fish sticks for 3 minutes.
- When done, sprinkle lemon zest over the fish sticks, drizzle with lemon juice and then sprinkle parsley over the top.
- Serve the fish sticks with your favorite sauce, which you can prepare from the 'Sauces, Dips, and Dressing' section.

Kale Chips

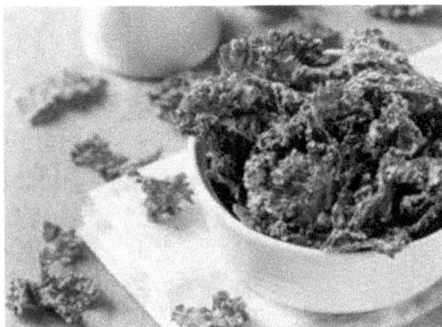

Nutritional Information per Serving

Calories: 176 calories
Fat: 16g
Sat. Fat: 3g
Carbohydrates: 4.4g
Protein: 3.4g
Fiber: 2.4g

Prep Time: 10 minutes | Cook Time: 30 minutes | Servings: 4

Ingredients

- 8 cups kale leaves
- 2 teaspoons lemon zest
- ½ teaspoon salt
- 2 teaspoons Italian seasoning

- ½ teaspoon ground black pepper
- 4 tablespoons olive oil
- 4 tablespoons grated parmesan cheese, low-fat

Directions

- Switch on the oven, then set it to 350 degrees F and let it preheat.
- Take a large baking sheet, line it with baking paper, and then spread the kale leaves in a single layer.
- Season kale leaves with salt, black pepper, lemon zest, and parmesan cheese, drizzle with oil, toss until mixed, and then massage the leaves for 2 minutes.
- Place the prepared baking sheet containing kale leaves into the oven and bake for 15 minutes until crisp, turning halfway.
- When done, let the kale leaves rest until crisp further and repeat with the remaining kale leaves.

Vegetable Chips

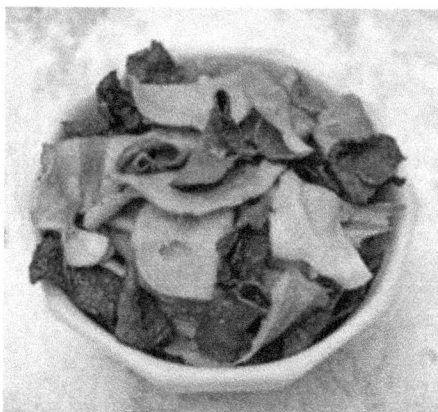

Nutritional Information per Serving

Calories: 100 calories
Fat: 5g
Sat. Fat: 1g
Carbohydrates: 14g
Protein: 2g
Fiber: 6g

Prep Time: 15 minutes | Cook Time: 30 minutes | Servings: 4

Ingredients

- 2 medium beetroots, peeled
- 1 medium rutabaga, peeled
- 1 large zucchini, peeled
- 1 small sweet potato, peeled

- 1 teaspoon salt
- 1 teaspoon garlic powder
- ½ teaspoon ground black pepper
- ½ cup olive oil

Directions

- Switch on the oven, then set it to 450 degrees F and let it preheat.
- Meanwhile, take 2 large rimmed baking sheets, line them with foil and then brush them with oil, set them aside until required.
- Peel the vegetables, cut them into 1/8-inch-thick slices, and then spread them in a single layer on the prepared baking sheets.
- Brush the top of vegetable slices with the remaining oil and then sprinkle with garlic powder, salt, and black pepper.
- Place the prepared baking sheets into the oven and then bake for 30 minutes until nicely browned and crisp, turning halfway.
- Serve the vegetable chips with your favorite dip, which you can prepare from the 'Sauces, Dips, and Dressing' section.

Chapter 9

Dinner

Cod with Tomatoes and Olives

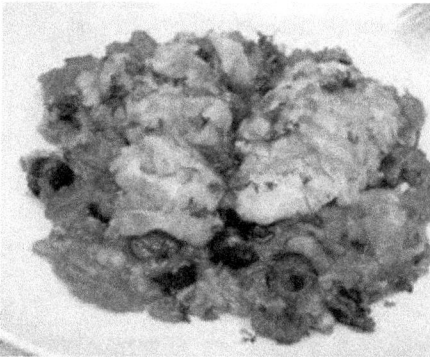

Nutritional Information per Serving

Calories: 256 calories
Fat: 16g
Sat. Fat: 3g
Carbohydrates: 6g
Protein: 24g
Fiber: 3g

Prep Time: 10 minutes | Cook Time: 15 minutes | Servings: 4; 1 plate per serving

Ingredients

- 1 pound fillet of cod, deboned
- ¼ cup basil leaves, chopped
- 10 ounces baby spinach, fresh
- 1 teaspoon salt
- 1/3 cup kalamata olives, sliced
- ½ teaspoon ground black pepper
- ¼ cup sun-dried tomatoes, sliced, packed in oil

- ¼ cup parsley leaves, chopped
- 6 pepperoncini, sliced
- ½ teaspoon red pepper flakes
- 2 tablespoons olive oil
- ¼ cup pine nuts
- ¼ cup crumbled feta cheese, low-fat

Directions

- Switch on the oven, then set it to 400 degrees F and let it preheat.
- Take a baking dish about the size of a fish fillet, grease it with 1 tablespoon oil, scatter spinach leaves in the bottom and then top with the fillet, skin-side-down.
- Sprinkle salt and black pepper over the fillet, drizzle with remaining, top with tomatoes, olives, nuts, and pepperoncini, and then sprinkle with the red pepper flakes.
- Sprinkle basil leaves and parsley leaves over the fillet, and bake the fish for 10 minutes.
- Then sprinkle feta cheese over the fish, continue baking for 5 minutes and then serve.

Grilled Sea Bass

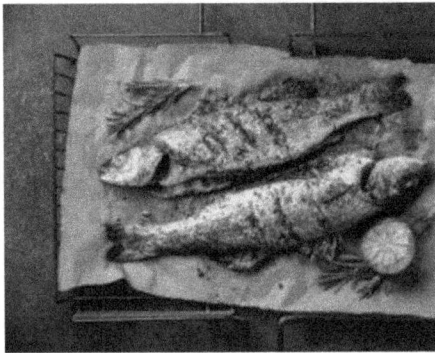

Nutritional Information per Serving

Calories: 305 calories
Fat: 15g
Sat. Fat: 3g
Carbohydrates: 1g
Protein: 40g
Fiber: 0g

Prep Time: 25 minutes | Cook Time: 20 minutes | Servings: 4

Ingredients

- 2 whole sea bass, about 1 ½
- ¼ teaspoon ground black pepper

- pounds, cleaned
- 1 ¼ teaspoon salt
- 2 tablespoons lemon juice
- 1 tablespoon chopped oregano leaves
- 1 tablespoon lemon zest

- 3 tablespoons olive oil
- 1 teaspoon ground coriander
- 2 large sprigs of oregano
- 1 lemon, cut into wedges

Directions

- Take a small bowl, place lemon zest, coriander, oregano, and ¼ teaspoon salt, pour in lemon juice and oil, and then stir until mixed.
- Pat dry the sea bass with paper towels, make three cuts into each fish and then season with black pepper and remaining salt.
- Stuff each fish with oregano sprigs and lemon wedges and arrange them into a baking dish.
- Rub the fishes with half of the prepared oil mixture and let them rest for 15 minutes.
- Meanwhile, take a griddle pan, grease it with oil, place it over medium-high heat and let it preheat.
- Place the prepared fish on the griddle pan and then cook for 15 to 20 minutes until fork-tender, turning halfway.
- When done, transfer fish to a cutting board, make a cut along the backbone of the fish, use a spatula to lift out the backbone and ribs, and discard them.
- Repeat with the other fish, transfer fish to a plate, drizzle the remaining oil mixture on top and then serve.

Shrimp in Garlic Sauce

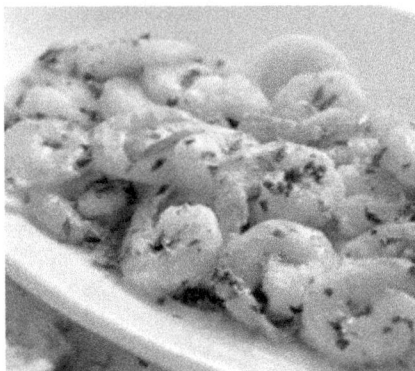

Nutritional Information per Serving

Calories: 268.5 calories
Fat: 12.1g
Sat. Fat: 1.6g
Carbohydrates: 1.8g
Protein: 37.5g
Fiber: 0.75g

Prep Time: 5 minutes | Cook Time: 10 minutes | Servings: 4

Ingredients

- 1 ½ pound shrimps, peeled, deveined
- 6 teaspoons minced garlic
- 1 ½ teaspoon salt
- 1 ½ tablespoon lemon juice
- ¾ teaspoon ground black pepper
- ½ teaspoon red pepper flakes
- 1/3 tablespoon vegetable broth
- 3 tablespoons olive oil

Directions

- Take a large skillet pan, place it over medium heat, add oil and when hot, add garlic and cook for 1 minute until fragrant.
- Add shrimps, season with salt, black pepper, and red pepper flakes, pour in the lemon juice, stir until mixed, and then cook for 1 minute.
- Then switch heat to the low level, pour in the broth, stir until just mixed, and then cook for 5 to 8 minutes until the shrimps turn pink.
- Serve shrimps alone or over the cooked whole-wheat pasta.

Greek Turkey Burgers

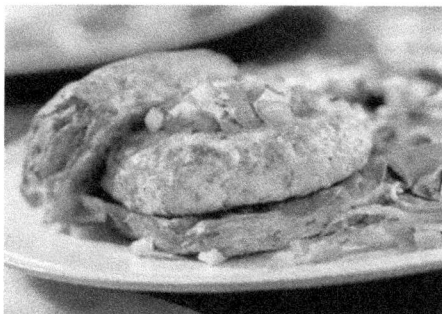

Nutritional Information per Serving

Calories: 376 calories
Fat: 17g
Sat. Fat: 6.2g
Carbohydrates: 28.5g
Protein: 30g
Fiber: 5g

Prep Time: 15 minutes | Cook Time: 10 minutes | Servings: 4; 1 burger per serving

Ingredients

- 1 cup chopped spinach, fresh or thawed if frozen
- 1 pound ground turkey, extra-lean
- ½ teaspoon garlic powder
- ¼ teaspoon salt
- ½ teaspoon dried oregano
- ¼ teaspoon ground black pepper
- 1 cup chopped spinach, fresh or thawed if frozen
- 1 pound ground turkey, extra-lean
- ½ teaspoon garlic powder
- ¼ teaspoon salt
- ½ teaspoon dried oregano
- ¼ teaspoon ground black pepper

Directions

- Squeeze the spinach to remove excess water and then place it in a large bowl.
- Add ground turkey, salt, black pepper, oregano, garlic powder, and feta cheese, stir until well combined, and then shape the mixture into four evenly sized patties.
- Take a griddle pan, grease it with oil, place it over medium-high heat and let it preheat.
- Arrange the prepared patties on the griddle pan and then cook for 5 to 8 minutes per side until golden brown and thoroughly cooked.
- Assemble the burgers and for this, take a bottom half of the hamburger, place a turkey patty on it and then spoon 1 tablespoon of the prepared tzatziki sauce on it.

- •
  - Top with 3 slices of cucumber, 2 onion rings, and then cover with the top half of the hamburger.
  - Prepare the remaining burgers in the same manner and then serve.

Grilled Chicken Kabobs

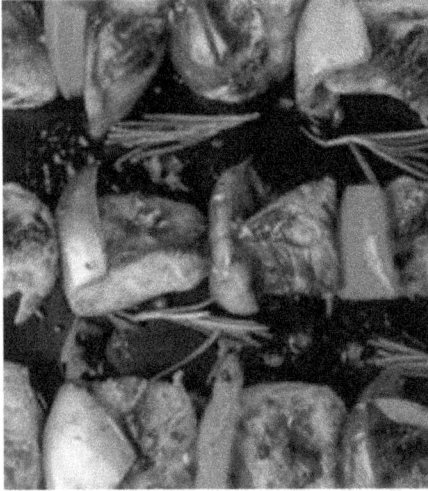

Nutritional Information per Serving

Calories: 296 calories
Fat: 20.4g
Sat. Fat: 3g
Carbohydrates: 12.2g
Protein: 17.6g
Fiber: 2.8g

Prep Time: 2 hours and 15 minutes | Cook Time: 20 minutes | Servings: 24 skewers; 6 skewers per serving

Ingredients

- 4 pounds chicken breasts, boneless, skinless, 1 ½-inch cubed
- 2 medium green bell peppers, cored, cut into 1 ½-inch piece
- 2 large white onions, peeled, sliced
- 2 medium red bell peppers, cored, cut into 1 ½-inch piece
- 2 teaspoons ground nutmeg
- 2 teaspoons dried thyme
- 2 teaspoons ground black pepper
- 3 teaspoons paprika
- 25 cloves of garlic, peeled, minced
- 1 cup olive oil
- 2 medium red onions, cored, cut into 1 ½-inch piece
- 5 lemons, juiced
- Tahini sauce as needed for

- 3 teaspoons salt
- ½ teaspoon ground cardamom

serving (prepare from the 'Sauces, Dips, and Dressing' section)

Directions

- Prepare a spice mix and for this, take a small bowl, place ¼ teaspoon each of salt and black pepper along with thyme, cardamom, paprika, and nutmeg and then stir until mixed.
- Take a large bowl, place chicken pieces in it, add prepared spice mix, and then toss well until coated.
- Add white onion slices and garlic, drizzle with lemon juice and oil, toss until coated, cover the bowl with its lid, place it in the refrigerator and let it rest for 4 hours.
- When ready to cook, take a griddle pan, grease it with oil, place it over medium-high heat and let it preheat.
- Thread chicken pieces, red onion, and bell pepper slices onto wooden skewers, arrange the skewers on the griddle pan, and cook for 10 to 12 minutes or more until thoroughly cooked.
- Serve the chicken skewers with tahini sauce.

Sweet and Sour Chicken

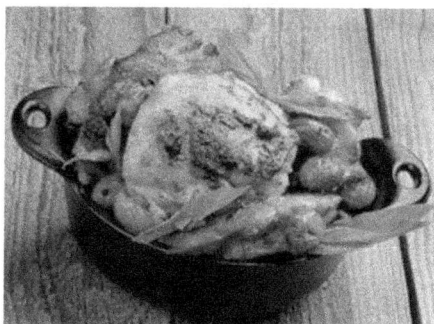

Nutritional Information per Serving

Calories: 375 calories
Fat: 11g
Sat. Fat: 2g
Carbohydrates: 30g
Protein: 38g
Fiber: 5g

Prep Time: 10 minutes | Cook Time: 35 minutes | Servings: 4; 1 plate per serving

Ingredients

- 2 pounds chicken thighs, boneless, skinless
- ¾ cup figs, halved
- 1 tablespoon minced garlic
- 2 teaspoons cornstarch
- ¼ teaspoon salt

- 2 teaspoons coconut sugar
- 2 teaspoons olive oil
- ¼ cup red wine vinegar
- ½ cup chicken broth
- ¼ cup salad olives, stuffed
- 5 ounces baby arugula, fresh

Directions

- Take a large skillet pan, place it over medium-high heat, add oil, and when hot, add chicken thighs.
- Season them with salt and then cook for 17 to 20 minutes until the chicken turns nicely golden brown and thoroughly cooked, covering the pan with its lid.
- When done, transfer the chicken thighs to a plate, add minced garlic into the skillet pan and then cook for 30 seconds until fragrant.
- Meanwhile, take a medium bowl, pour in the broth and vinegar, and then whisk in sugar and cornstarch until blended.
- Pour the broth mixture into the skillet pan, stir well to loosen browned bits at the bottom of the pan, and then bring the sauce to a boil.
- Continue boiling the sauce for 1 minute or more until thickened to the desired level, add olives, chicken thighs, and figs and then cook for 3 to 4 minutes until thoroughly hot.
- Divide the arugula among four plates, top with the chicken and its sauce, and then serve.

Hasselback Caprese Chicken

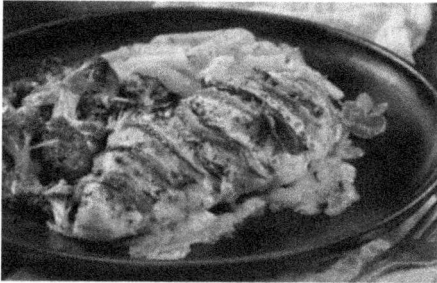

Nutritional Information per Serving

Calories: 311 calories
Fat: 15.9g
Sat. Fat: 5.9g
Carbohydrates: 9g
Protein: 32.6g
Fiber: 4.2g

Prep Time: 15 minutes | Cook Time: 25 minutes | Servings: 4

Ingredients

- 2 chicken breasts, skinless, boneless, each about 8 ounces
- 4 cups broccoli florets
- ½ teaspoon salt, divided
- 1 medium tomato, sliced
- ½ teaspoon ground black pepper, divided
- ¼ cup prepared pesto
- 2 tablespoons olive oil
- 3 ounces mozzarella cheese, halved, sliced, low-fat

Directions

- Switch on the oven, then set it to 375 degrees F and let it preheat.
- Meanwhile, prepare the chicken breasts and for this, make crosswise cuts in it, not all the way through, and at every ½ inch.
- Season each chicken breast with ¼ teaspoon each of salt and black pepper and then stuff the cuts in chicken breasts alternately with a tomato slice and cheese slice.
- Take a large bowl, place broccoli florets in it, add remaining salt and black pepper, drizzle with oil and then toss until coated.
- Take a large baking sheet, place the prepared chicken breasts on one side of the baking sheet, and then scatter broccoli florets on the other side of the baking sheet.

- Bake the prepared chicken breasts and broccoli florets for 25 minutes or more until chicken has thoroughly cooked and broccoli turns tender, stirring broccoli halfway.
- When done, cut each chicken breast in half and then serve each chicken breast piece with one-fourth of the roasted broccoli florets.

Lentil, Chickpea and Tomato Soup

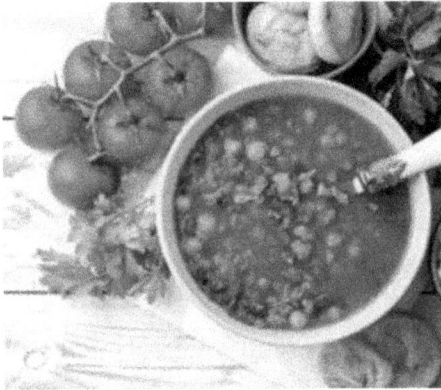

Nutritional Information per Serving

Calories: 291 calories
Fat: 9g
Sat. Fat: 1.5g
Carbohydrates: 42g
Protein: 12g
Fiber: 13.5g

Prep Time: 10 minutes | Cook Time: 35 minutes | Servings: 4

Ingredients

- ½ cup green lentils, uncooked, rinsed
- ¼ cup white whole-wheat flour
- 1 large white onion, peeled, sliced
- 1 stick of celery, chopped
- 1 cup cooked chickpeas
- 1 cup cilantro leaves
- 4 tomatoes, peeled
- 1 cup parsley leaves
- 1 teaspoon salt
- ½ cup whole-wheat thin pasta, broken in quarters
- 1 teaspoon turmeric powder
- 1 teaspoon ground black pepper
- ½ teaspoon ginger powder
- ½ piece of vegetable bouillon cube, salted
- 2 tablespoons olive oil
- 4 tablespoons tomato paste
- 6 ¼ cups water

Directions

- Plug in a food processor, add onion, celery, tomatoes, and ½ cup each of parsley and cilantro, and then pulse until smooth.
- Pour the mixture into a large pot, add 2 cups of water, place the pot over high heat and then bring it to a boil.
- Add ginger, lentils, bouillon cube, tomato paste, and olive oil, stir in salt, black pepper, and turmeric and then bring the soup to boil.
- Then switch heat to the low level, simmer the soup for 10 minutes, add pasta and chickpeas, pour in 4 cups water, bring the soup to boil, and then simmer for 5 minutes.
- Meanwhile, place flour in a blender, pour in the remaining water, and then pulse until smooth.
- After 5 minutes, slowly pour the flour mixture into the pot, stirring continuously, and then simmer for another 5 minutes.
- When done, add remaining cilantro and parsley leaves, taste to adjust seasoning, and then remove the pot from heat.
- Ladle the soup among 4 bowls and then serve.

Greek Red Lentil Soup

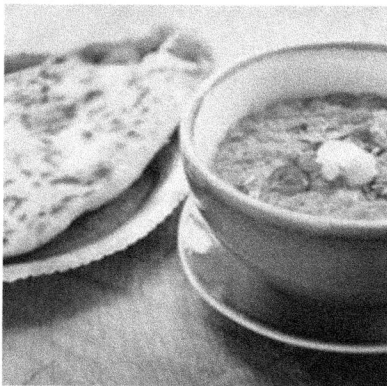

Nutritional Information per Serving

Calories: 293.3 calories
Fat: 4.5g
Sat. Fat: 1.2g
Carbohydrates: 47.4g
Protein: 15.8g
Fiber: 9.4g

Prep Time: 10 minutes | Cook Time: 30 minutes | Servings: 4; 1 bowl per serving

Ingredients

- 1 medium white onion, peeled, chopped
- ¾ cup crushed tomatoes
- 1 medium carrot, peeled, chopped
- 1 tablespoon minced garlic
- 2 teaspoons dried oregano
- 1 ½ cups red lentils, uncooked, rinsed, drained
- 1 teaspoon ground cumin
- ½ teaspoon dried rosemary
- 1 teaspoon salt
- ½ teaspoon red pepper flakes
- 2 bay leaves
- ½ of a lemon, zested
- 2 tablespoons olive oil
- 1 lemon, juiced
- 4 cups vegetable broth
- 4 tablespoons parsley leaves
- 4 tablespoons crumbled feta cheese, low-fat

Directions

- Take a large pot, place it over medium-high heat, add oil, and when hot, add onion, garlic, and carrots, and then cook for 4 minutes until vegetables begin to soften.
- Add oregano, cumin, oregano, rosemary, red pepper flakes, and bay leaves, and then cook for 1 minute until fragrant.
- Add lentils and tomatoes, pour in the broth, stir in salt and then bring the soup to a boil.
- Then switch heat to medium level and simmer the soup for 15 to 20 minutes until thoroughly cooked, covering the pot with its lid.
- When lentils have cooked, remove the pot from heat and then pulse it using an immersion blender until smooth and creamy.
- Return the pot over medium heat, cook for 3 to 4 minutes until thoroughly hot, and then stir in parsley, lemon zest, and juice.
- Divide the soup evenly among four bowls, drizzle with oil, top with feta cheese and then serve.

Greek Pasta

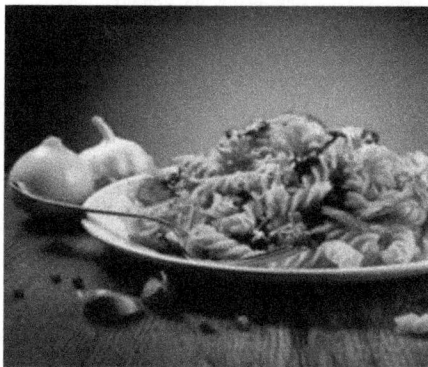

Nutritional Information per Serving

Calories: 308.3 calories
Fat: 8.7g
Sat. Fat: 3.1g
Carbohydrates: 40.4g
Protein: 17.1g
Fiber: 6g

Prep Time: 10 minutes | Cook Time: 25 minutes | Servings: 4

Ingredients

- 2 cups whole-wheat pasta
- 2 links of cooked chicken sausage, sliced into rounds
- ¾ cup diced white onion
- ½ teaspoon minced garlic
- 3 cups baby spinach
- 3 tablespoons chopped pitted Kalamata olives
- 1 ½ tablespoon olive oil
- 4 tablespoons crumbled feta cheese, low-fat
- 6 ounces canned tomato sauce, no-salt-added
- 3 tablespoons chopped basil

Directions

- Prepare the pasta, and for this, take a large pot half full with water, place it over medium-high heat and then bring it to a boil.
- Add the pasta, cook it for 8 to 10 minutes until tender, then drain it well and reserve ½ cup of a cooking liquid, set aside until required.
- Then take a large skillet pan, place it over medium-high heat, add oil, and when hot, add onion, sausage slices, and garlic, stir until mixed, and then cook for 4 to 6 minutes until onion begins to brown.

- Add the cooked pasta along with spinach, olives, and tomato sauce, stir until just mixed, and then cook for 3 to 5 minutes until spinach wilts and the sauce begins to bubble.
- Stir in basil leaves and feta cheese, then divide the prepared pasta evenly among four plates and serve.

Italian Minestrone Soup

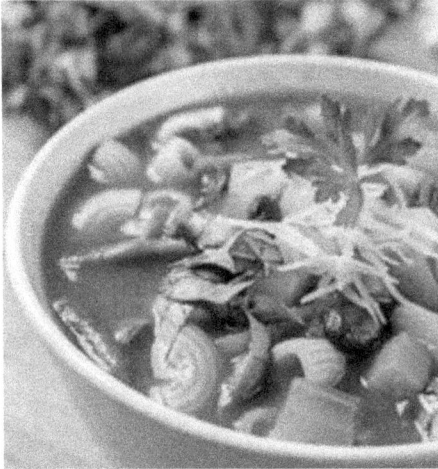

Nutritional Information per Serving

Calories: 301.7 calories
Fat: 9.3g
Sat. Fat: 2.5g
Carbohydrates: 39.7g
Protein: 14.8g
Fiber: 9.4g

Prep Time: 10 minutes | Cook Time: 40 minutes | Servings: 4; 1 bowl per serving

Ingredients

- 2 cups cooked small whole-wheat pasta
- 1 cup green beans, ends trimmed, cut into 1-inch pieces
- 1 small white onion, peeled, chopped
- 2 tablespoons minced garlic
- 15 ounces cooked kidney beans
- 2 medium carrots, peeled,

- 1 teaspoon salt
- ½ teaspoon ground black pepper
- 1 teaspoon paprika
- 2 sprigs of thyme
- ½ teaspoon dried rosemary
- ¼ cup chopped parsley
- 1 bay leaf
- ¼ cup olive oil
- ¼ cup basil leaves
- 6 cups vegetable broth
- 4 tablespoons grated Parmesan

cheese, low-fat

- chopped
- 1 large zucchini, ends trimmed, diced
- 2 celery stalks, diced
- 15 ounces crushed tomatoes

Directions

- Take a large pot, place it over medium-high heat, add oil, and when hot, add onion, celery, and carrots, and then cook for 5 minutes until vegetables begin to soften.
- Stir in garlic, cook for 1 minute, add green beans and zucchini, and then stir in rosemary, paprika, and ¼ teaspoon each of salt and black pepper until combined.
- Add tomatoes, bay leaf, and thyme, pour in the broth, bring it to a boil, then switch heat to medium-low level and simmer the soup for 20 minutes, covering the pot with its lid.
- Add kidney beans, continue cooking for 10 minutes and then stir in basil and parsley.
- Then add the cooked pasta, simmer for 2 to 3 minutes until thoroughly hot, and then remove the bay leaf.
- Taste the soup to adjust seasoning, remove the pot from heat, divide the soup evenly among four bowls and then serve.

Roasted Tomato and Basil Soup

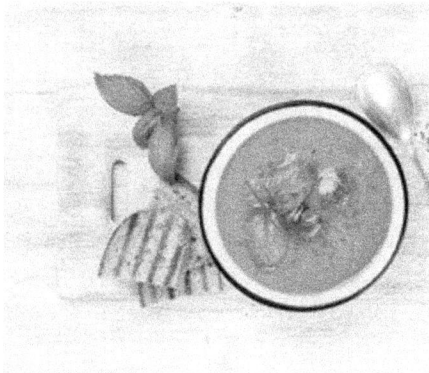

Nutritional Information per Serving

Calories: 322 calories
Fat: 16.8g
Sat. Fat: 3.1g
Carbohydrates: 33.4g
Protein: 9.3g
Fiber: 6.4g

Prep Time: 20 minutes | Cook Time: 1 hour | Servings: 4; 1 bowl per serving

Ingredients

- 2 pounds tomatoes, halved
- 2 medium white onions, chopped
- 1 teaspoon salt
- 4 cloves of garlic, peeled, minced
- 2/3 teaspoon dried thyme
- 2 medium carrots, peeled, diced
- 2/3 teaspoon dried oregano
- 2/3 cup crushed tomatoes
- ¾ teaspoon ground black pepper
- 1/3 teaspoon ground cumin

- 1-ounce fresh basil leaves
- 1/3 teaspoon paprika
- 4 tablespoons olive oil
- 1 ¾ cup water

For Serving:

- 8 slices of whole-wheat French baguette, each about 1-inch thick
- 1 ½ teaspoon minced garlic
- 1 ½ teaspoon Italian herb seasoning
- ¾ cup butter, unsalted, melted
- ¼ teaspoon ground red pepper

Directions

- Switch on the oven, then set it to 450 degrees F and let it preheat.
- Meanwhile, take a large bowl, place carrot pieces and tomato halves in it, drizzle with 2 tablespoons of oil, season with ¼ teaspoon each of salt and black pepper, and then toss until combined.
- Take a large baking sheet, spread the vegetable mixture in a single layer, and then roast for 30 minutes until tender, stirring halfway.
- When done, let the vegetables cool for 10 minutes, transfer them to a blender, add ¼ cup water and then pulse until blended.
- Take a large pot, place it over medium-high heat, add remaining oil and when hot, add onions and then cook for 3 minutes or until beginning to tender.
- Add garlic, cook for 1 minute until fragrant, add the blended tomato-carrot mixture, crushed tomatoes, basil, cumin, paprika, thyme, and remaining salt, black pepper, and water, and then stir until mixed.
- Bring the soup to boil, then switch heat to low level and simmer for 20 to 30 minutes until soup has reached to desired consistency, covering the pot part-way with its lid.
- While the soup cooks, grill the bread slices, and for this, place the butter in a medium heatproof bowl and then microwave for 1 to 2 minutes until melted, stirring every 30 seconds.

- Add Italian herb seasoning, garlic, and red pepper into the melted butter and then stir until combined.
- Take a griddle pan, place it over medium-high heat and let it preheat.
- Working on one baguette slice at a time, dip both sides in the prepared butter mixture or brush the butter mixture generously on both pieces of bread and then place it on the griddle pan.
- Add more buttered bread slices in the griddle pan until filled and then grill for 2 to 3 minutes per side until nicely golden brown and developed grill marks.
- When done, divide the tomato soup evenly among four bowls, drizzle some more olive oil on top and then serve each bowl with 2 toasted slices of whole-wheat French baguette.

Chapter 10

Desserts

Olive Oil Gelato

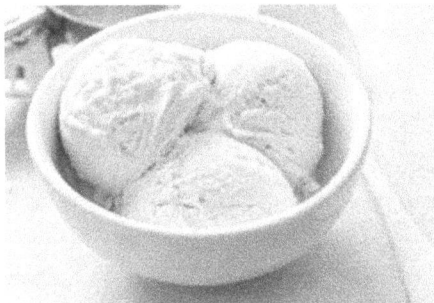

Nutritional Information per Serving

Calories: 234 calories
Fat: 18.4g
Sat. Fat: 4.2g
Carbohydrates: 14g
Protein: 2.9g
Fiber: 0.3g

Prep Time: 7 hours | Cook Time: 15 minutes | Servings: 4; 1 bowl per serving

Ingredients

- ¾ cup coconut sugar
- 4 egg yolks, at room temperature
- 1/8 teaspoon salt
- ¼ cup and 2 tablespoons water
- ¼ cup olive oil
- ¾ cup coconut milk, unsweetened, low-fat

Directions

- Take a medium pot, pour in the water and milk, and then stir in salt and sugar until mixed.
- Place the pot over medium heat and then cook for 3 to 5 minutes until bubbles form around the edges of the pot.
- Meanwhile, take a large bowl, fill it with ice, place another bowl on the ice and set it aside until required.

- Take a separate large bowl, place egg yolks in it and then whisk until frothy.
- Then whisk in the milk mixture in a steady stream until combined, and then pour this mixture into the pot.
- Switch heat to a low level and cook the custard until it has thickened enough to coat the back of a spoon, or its temperature reaches 185 degrees F, stirring continuously.
- Then immediately spoon the custard into the bowl placed over ice, and then stir the custard until cooled.
- When cooled, cover the custard bowl with its lid, place it into the refrigerator and let it chill overnight.
- Then whisk oil into the custard in a steady stream until smooth, cover the bowl with its lid, and place it in the refrigerator for 6 hours, stirring every 1 hour.
- You can also churn the custard in an ice cream maker.
- When ready to eat, let the gelato rest for 15 minutes at room temperature, scoop it into bowls, and then serve.

Chocolate Avocado Mousse

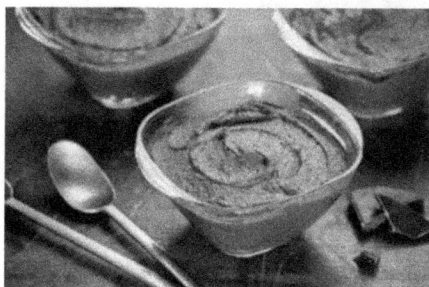

Nutritional Information per Serving

Calories: 240 calories
Fat: 12.7g
Sat. Fat: 2g
Carbohydrates: 28.1g
Protein: 2.9g
Fiber: 9.8g

Prep Time: 35 minutes | Cook Time: 0 minutes | Servings: 4; 1 bowl per serving

Ingredients

- 2 avocados, peeled, pitted
- 6 tablespoons date syrup
- 1 banana, peeled
- ½ teaspoon vanilla extract,

- ¼ cup cocoa powder, unsweetened
- 1 tablespoon almond butter, unsalted
- 2 tablespoons almond milk, low-

- unsweetened

- fat, unsweetened
- Berries as needed for topping

Directions

- Peel the bananas, cut them into pieces, and add them to a blender.
- Cut avocado into slices, add to the blender along with almond butter, date syrup, vanilla, and milk, and then pulse until combined.
- Divide the mousse evenly among four bowls, place them in the refrigerator and let them chill for 30 minutes or until required.
- When ready to eat, top the mousse with berries or favorite fruits and then serve.

Rice Pudding with Almond Milk

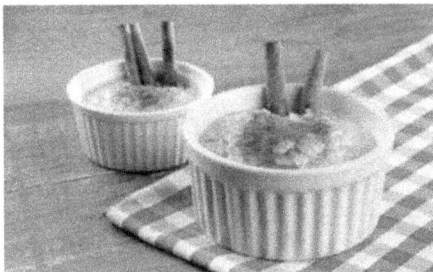

Nutritional Information per Serving

Calories: 257 calories
Fat: 6.3g
Sat. Fat: 0.7g
Carbohydrates: 41.7g
Protein: 8.3g
Fiber: 3.6g

Prep Time: 10 minutes | Cook Time: 30 minutes | Servings: 4; 1 bowl per serving

Ingredients

- 1/3 cup Medjool dates, pitted
- 1/3 cup whole raisins
- ¾ cup brown rice, uncooked
- ½ teaspoon vanilla extract, unsweetened
- ¼ toasted and chopped, sliced almonds

- ¼ teaspoon almond extract, unsweetened
- 1/8 teaspoon ground cinnamon
- 3 cups almond milk, vanilla flavor, unsweetened, low-fat
- 1/3 cup boiling water

Directions

- Prepare the date syrup and for this, take a medium bowl, place dates in it, pour in the boiling water, and let them soak for 15 minutes.
- Then transfer the dates with water into a food processor and pulse until smooth, set aside until required.
- Take a medium saucepan, place rice in it, pour in the milk, and then bring the mixture to a boil.
- Switch heat to medium-low level, simmer the rice for 20 to 30 minutes until rice has absorbed all the milk, stirring occasionally.
- Then add almonds, raisins, cinnamon, prepared date syrup, and vanilla, and almond extract and stir until mixed.
- Divide the pudding evenly among four bowls and then serve.

Vanilla Baked Pears

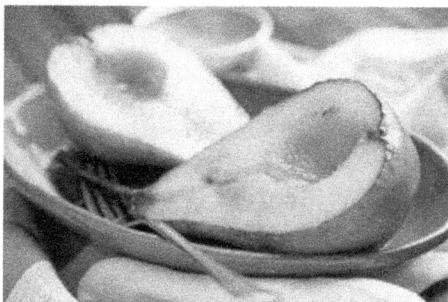

Nutritional Information per Serving

Calories: 216 calories
Fat: 0.5g
Sat. Fat: 0.25g
Carbohydrates: 50.6g
Protein: 2.1g
Fiber: 6.6g

Prep Time: 10 minutes | Cook Time: 25 minutes | Servings: 4; 2 pear halves per serving

Ingredients

- 4 medium pears
- ½ cup date syrup
- ¼ teaspoon ground cinnamon
- 1 teaspoon vanilla extract, unsweetened
- 4 tablespoons Greek yogurt, low-fat

Directions

- Switch on the oven, then set it to 375 degrees F and let it preheat.
- Meanwhile, cut each pear in half, remove its core using a small cookie scoop, and then cut a little piece from the bottom to make pear halves stand upright on a baking sheet.
- Take a large baking sheet, arrange pear halves in it cut-side-up and then sprinkle with cinnamon.
- Take a small bowl, place vanilla extract and date syrup in it, whisk until combined, and then drizzle over the prepared pear halves, reserving 2 tablespoons of the syrup for later use.
- Place the prepared baking sheet into the oven and bake the pears for 25 minutes until the edges turn golden brown.
- When done, drizzle the reserved maple syrup over the roasted pears and then divide pear halves among four plates, 2 pear halves per plate.
- Add 1 tablespoon yogurt to each plate and then serve.

Strawberry Popsicles

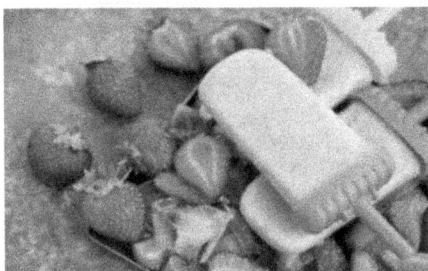

Nutritional Information per Serving

Calories: 38 calories
Fat: 0.6g
Sat. Fat: 0.05g
Carbohydrates: 6.9g
Protein: 0.6g
Fiber: 1.9g

Prep Time: 4 hours and 10 minutes | Cook Time: 0 minutes | Servings: 4; 1 popsicle per serving

Ingredients

- 2 ½ cups strawberries, fresh, rinsed
- ½ cup almond milk, unsweetened, low-fat

Directions

- Wash the berries and using a small sharp knife, remove the hull from each berry and discard it.
- Place the strawberries into a blender, pour in the milk, and then pulse until smooth.
- Divide the berries mixture evenly among the four popsicle molds, place a stick into each popsicle and then place the popsicle molds in a freezer.
- Let the popsicle freeze for a minimum of 4 hours or until firm and then serve.

Coconut, Tahini, and Cashew Bars

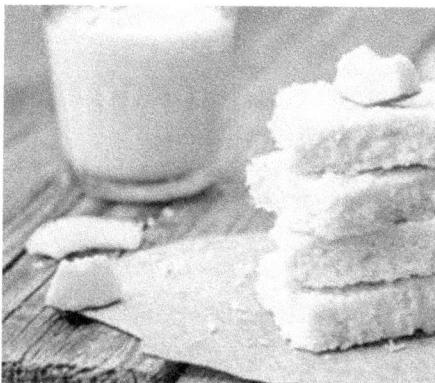

Nutritional Information per Serving

Calories: 155 calories
Fat: 11.8g
Sat. Fat: 4.3g
Carbohydrates: 8.7g
Protein: 2.6g
Fiber: 1.6g

Prep Time: 35 minutes | Cook Time: 0 minutes | Servings: 8; 2 bars per serving

Ingredients

For the Base:

- 2 Medjool dates, pitted
- ⅛ teaspoon salt
- ¼ cup walnuts
- ½ tablespoon coconut oil
- 2 tablespoons cashews

For the Filling:

- ¼ cup dried coconut, unsweetened, more as needed for sprinkling
- ¼ cup cashew butter
- ¼ teaspoon ground cinnamon
- 2 tablespoons tahini (prepared from the 'Sauces, Dips, and Dressing' section)

- ¼ teaspoon salt
- ½ tablespoon coconut oil

Directions

- Take a small bowl, place the pitted dates in it, cover with warm water, and then let the dates rest for 5 minutes or more until softened.
- Then drain the dates, add them into the blender, add salt, nuts, oil, and cashews and then pulse until combined and the mixture resembles dough.
- Take a square bread pan, line it with a parchment sheet, spoon the date mixture in it, spread it evenly, then place the pan into a freezer and then let it rest for 10 minutes.
- Meanwhile, prepare the filling and for this, place all of its ingredients in a blender and then pulse until smooth.
- Spoon the prepared filling mixture into the prepared bread pan, spread it evenly, and then sprinkle some more coconut on top.
- Return the bread pan into the freezer and let it freeze for another 15 minutes.
- Then take out the crust by pulling it out using the parchment sheet and then cut the crust into 1-inch rectangle-sized bars.
- Transfer the bars into an air-tight container and store them in a freezer until ready to eat.

- ## Applesauce Oat Muffins

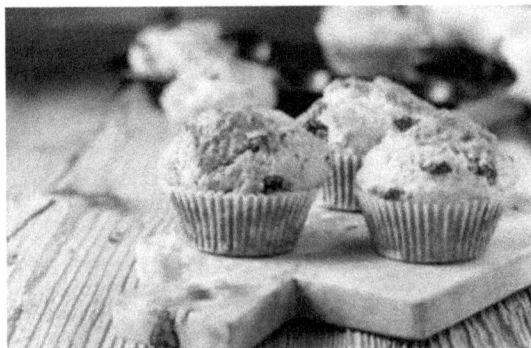

Nutritional Information per Serving

Calories: 196 calories
Fat: 1.1g
Sat. Fat: 0.3g
Carbohydrates: 24.6g
Protein: 23.5g
Fiber: 1.8g

Prep Time: 10 minutes | Cook Time: 20 minutes | Servings: 4 muffins; 1 muffin per serving

Ingredients

- ½ cup old-fashioned rolled oats
- 6 tablespoons whole-wheat flour
- ½ teaspoon baking powder
- ½ teaspoon ground cinnamon
- 3 tablespoons coconut sugar
- 1/3 teaspoon baking soda
- 1/8 teaspoon salt
- ½ cup applesauce, unsweetened
- 1 ½ tablespoon melted coconut oil
- 3 tablespoons almond milk, unsweetened, low-fat
- ½ teaspoon vanilla extract, unsweetened
- ¼ cup raisins
- ½ of a large egg

Directions

- Switch on the oven, then set it to 375 degrees F and let it preheat.
- Take 4 large silicone muffin cups, grease them with oil, and set aside until required.
- Take a medium bowl, place oats, sugar, egg, and coconut oil, pour in milk and applesauce and stir until well combined.
- Take another medium bowl, place whole-wheat flour in it, add salt, baking powder, cinnamon, baking soda, and raisins and then stir until mixed.
- Slowly stir in oats mixture until incorporated and then divide the batter evenly among four prepared silicone muffin cups.
- Place the prepared muffin cups in the oven and then bake for 15 to 20 minutes until firm and the top turns golden brown.
- When done, let the muffins cool in their cups for 10 minutes, then take them out and cool completely before serving.

Baked Apple Slices

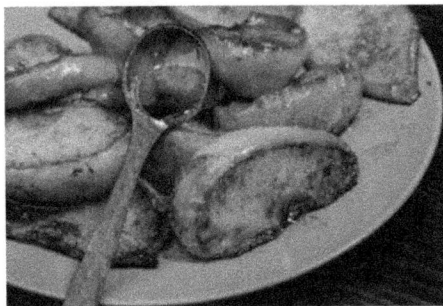

Nutritional Information
per Serving

Calories: 228 calories
Fat: 10.5g
Sat. Fat: 8g
Carbohydrates: 32g
Protein: 1g
Fiber: 3g

Prep Time: 10 minutes | Cook Time: 20 minutes | Servings: 4

Ingredients

- 4 large apples, unpeeled
- 4 teaspoons ground cinnamon

- 4 tablespoons cashew butter, unsalted, melted

Directions

- Switch on the oven, then set it to 400 degrees F and let it preheat.
- Meanwhile, take a square rimmed baking sheet about 8-inches, line it with a parchment sheet, and set it aside until required.
- Cut each apple in half, remove its core, and then slice each apple half into six pieces, each about ¼-inch thick.
- Scatter the apple pieces in a single layer, drizzle with melted butter, toss them until coated, and then spread the apple pieces in a single layer.
- Sprinkle 2 teaspoons of cinnamon on top of apple slices and then bake the apples for 10 minutes.
- Then flip the apple pieces, sprinkle the remaining cinnamon on top, and then continue baking for 10 minutes until apple slices turn tender and nicely golden brown.
- Serve straight away.

Chocolate Dipped Strawberries

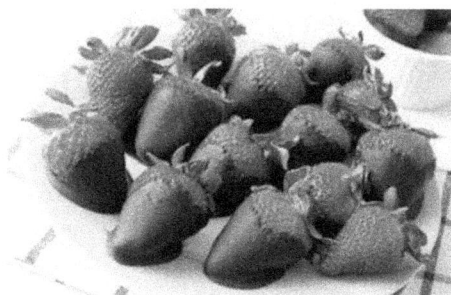

Nutritional Information per Serving

Calories: 235 calories
Fat: 16g
Sat. Fat: 6g
Carbohydrates: 18g
Protein: 4g
Fiber: 4g

Prep Time: 45 minutes | Cook Time: 2 minutes | Servings: 12 strawberries; 4 strawberries per serving

Ingredients

- 12 strawberries, fresh, rinsed
- 1 tablespoon cashew butter, unsalted
- 1 cup chocolate chips, unsweetened
- 1 teaspoon sesame seeds

Directions

- Take a medium heatproof bowl, place chocolate chips, and then microwave for 1 to 2 minutes until chocolate has melted, stirring every 30 seconds.
- Take a large baking sheet, line it with a parchment sheet, and set aside until required.
- Working on one strawberry at a time, hold it from its stem, and then dip it into the melted chocolate to coat it.
- Place the strawberry on the prepared baking sheet, sprinkle some sesame seeds on the coated strawberry and then repeat with the remaining berries.
- Place the prepared baking sheet containing berries in a refrigerator, let it rest for 40 minutes until chocolate has firmed, and then serve.

Watermelon and Mint Granita

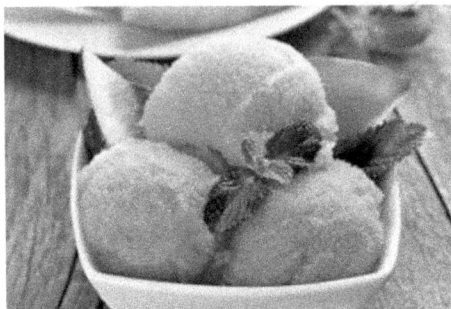

Nutritional Information per Serving

Calories: 168 calories
Fat: 0.4g
Sat. Fat: 0.04g
Carbohydrates: 39.2g
Protein: 1.2g
Fiber: 2.4g

Prep Time: 3 hours and 30 minutes | Cook Time: 0 minutes | Servings: 4; 1 bowl per serving

Ingredients

- 8 cups watermelon cubes, deseeded
- 3 limes, juiced
- 6 tablespoons coconut sugar
- 2 tablespoons mint leaves, chopped
- ½ teaspoon peppermint extract, unsweetened

Directions

- Place the watermelon pieces in a food processor and then pulse until smooth.
- Take a large bowl, place a fine sieve on it and then pass through the watermelon mixture and then discard the solids.
- Add lime juice into the collected watermelon mixture, add mint, sugar, and peppermint extract and then stir until sugar has dissolved.
- Take a 9-by-13 inches metal baking pan, pour the watermelon mixture in it, place it in the freezer and let it rest for 30 minutes.
- Remove the baking pan from the freezer, scrape granita using a fork, return it into the freezer for 3 hours, scrape granita every 30 minutes and then serve.

Peach Soup

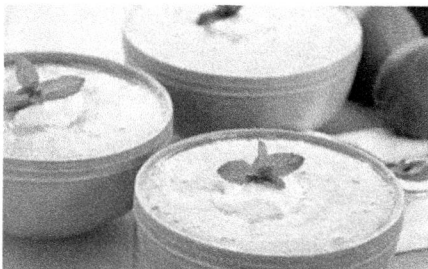

Nutritional Information per Serving

Calories: 258 calories
Fat: 17.2g
Sat. Fat: 4.3g
Carbohydrates: 21.3g
Protein: 4.5g
Fiber: 3.1g

Prep Time: 1 hour and 5 minutes | Cook Time: 0 minutes | Servings: 4

Ingredients

- 3 cups sliced peaches
- ¼ cup cucumber pieces, peeled
- ½ teaspoon salt
- 1 clove of garlic, peeled
- ¼ teaspoon ground black pepper
- ¼ cup green bell pepper pieces
- 2 tablespoons honey, raw
- ¼ cup balsamic vinegar
- 3 tablespoons goat cheese, low-fat, and more as needed for topping
- ¼ cup water
- ¼ cup olive oil and more as needed

Directions

- Place peaches, green bell pepper, and cucumber pieces in a blender, and then add garlic, salt, black pepper, honey, vinegar, and goat cheese.
- Pour in the water and oil, pulse until well combined, and then pour the soup into a large bowl.
- Taste it to adjust seasoning, then cover the soup bowl with its lid, place it in the refrigerator and let it rest for 1 hour until cold.
- When ready to eat, divide the soup evenly among four bowls, top with some goat cheese, drizzle with some oil and then serve.

Grilled Watermelon Salad

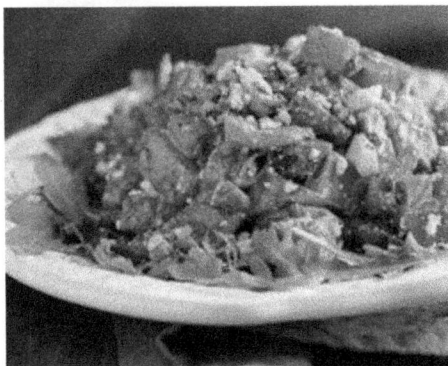

Nutritional Information per Serving

Calories: 171 calories
Fat: 7.05g
Sat. Fat: 2.4g
Carbohydrates: 20.4g
Protein: 5.4g
Fiber: 1.1g

Prep Time: 20 minutes | Cook Time: 8 minutes | Servings: 4; 1 bowl per serving

Ingredients

- 1 small watermelon
- 4 leaves of basil, chopped
- 1 lemon, juiced, zested
- 4 leaves of mint
- 1 tablespoon olive oil
- ½ cup grated parmesan cheese

Directions

- Prepare the watermelon and for this, cut it into quarters and then cut each piece into ½-inch thick triangles.
- Take a griddle pan, place it over medium-high heat and let it preheat until hot.
- Brush the watermelon triangle pieces with oil, arrange them on the griddle pan and then cook for 3 to 4 minutes per side or more until grill marks appear.
- When done, transfer the watermelon pieces to a plate, cool them for 10 minutes, peel the rind and then chop the watermelon flesh.
- Transfer the chopped watermelon to a medium bowl, add basil, mint, lemon juice and zest, and cheese, and then stir until combined.
- Divide the salad evenly among four bowls and then serve.

Leave a 1-click review!

Customer Reviews

★★★★★ 2
5.0 out of 5 stars ▾

5 star		100%
4 star		0%
3 star		0%
2 star		0%
1 star		0%

Share your thoughts with other customers

Write a customer review

See all verified purchase reviews ›

I would be incredibly grateful if you take just 60 seconds to write just a brief review on Amazon, even if it's just a few sentences.

https://www.amazon.com/review/create-review-asin=B09MHF2XQ1

Conclusion

O ur lives are short and fleeting and therefore, we have a responsibility to make it count. We owe it to us and to our bodies that work relentlessly to keep us alive and healthy. We should not return all the unhealthy compounds in response to the healthy equilibrium that our biological system tries to maintain every single second of the day. Take a seat and think how unjust we have been to our bodies. It will fill your eyes in tears because millions and trillions of cells work together to keep us alive and healthy. Is that how we are returning the favor? We are living in times where we are constantly taught to work longer and harder.

Practicing a lifestyle like that gives us no time to think about what we eat to keep us going. We barely get enough time to stop and think about what needs to be changed in our eating patterns or what steps we need to take to adopt a new way of eating food. After juggling various diets, I finally understood that our food directly links with how efficiently we function in society, and I realized it when I switched to the Mediterranean diet. That's why this book, "Mediterranean Diet for Beginners," is a personal endeavor to make people realize that it is about time we eat healthily and give back to our bodies. By retreating to a healthy and prosperous living by transitioning to a Mediterranean diet, we can enjoy the perks of good health and tastes of nutritious food.

The Mediterranean diet is more than just what meets the eye. It is a way of living and loving to eat, and this diet is a prime instance of what a healthy diet regime should be. It allows the consumption of healthy and nutritious food coupled with sufficient exercise for a balanced life. The Mediterranean diet has been the favorite research area for nutrition scientists for decades, and every time, they end up discovering more benefits that further confirm that this diet should be the only standard healthy diet pattern for people to follow.

As mentioned previously, the discovery of the Mediterranean diet by Ancel Keys unlocked the door for the entire world to see how food impacts the quality of our lives. In addition, he unveiled the relationship between eating healthy and living longer. He also strived to make people understand the link between diet and severe health complications. Briefly speaking, the Mediterranean diet has been researched countless times on different population samples, healthy and ill alike. The results have further confirmed that it is the best regimen to ever exist. On a Mediterranean diet, health is defined in different ways. It does not limit health by being alive and able to work long hours without collapsing. Instead, it associates being healthy with aspects like what and how you eat, what kind of people you share meals with, how you utilize your free time, and lastly, how frequently you exercise? When your life lacks any of the listed components, you tend to suffer mentally, physically, and emotionally. All these factors combined, make up the basic principles of the Mediterranean diet.

And being on a Mediterranean diet is like a stroke of warmth on a cold winter evening, and the warmth comes from eating with your loved ones, being in their heartwarming presence. The Mediterranean diet treats meal times as social events, where all the family members should gather at a dining table and enjoy their food together. So, do not treat the Mediterranean diet like a typical diet regimen. Instead, consider it like committing to the Mediterranean culture where eating healthy food is prized and valued, where meals are prepared with love and shared with people we care about.

As an author and a body fat expert with long experience of the Mediterranean diet, I have tried my very best to deliver information through this ebook about the Mediterranean way of life and potential benefits, backed by authentic scientific studies. In addition, we learned how to shop for the ingredients, so if you make up your mind to transition to the Mediterranean diet, you should know what ingredients to shop for and from where. You can start by making small changes because even the smallest ones make up a huge difference in the long term. Besides, now you know how to swap processed foods and replace them with healthy and more wholesome and nutritious foods. By now, you have learned that following the Mediterranean diet involves eating lots of fresh produce such as fruits, vegetables, specified types of meat, and little to moderate consumption of red wine.

You have also learned what kind of fats you can consume or use for cooking; for instance, extra virgin olive oil is commonly used. Moreover, after reading this ebook, you have realized that following a Mediterranean diet is more about choosing to live healthy rather than solely losing weight. In addition, the section on meal portions and sizes is there to assist you in cooking calculated portions of meals so that no amount of food is wasted. Finally, by cooking the recipes shared in this ebook, you can invite friends over and share some of the best dinners filled with laughs, good people, and scrumptious foods.

If you find this book fun in exploring the diverse taste of the Mediterranean diet, please do share this experience by leaving your feedback on Amazon. Your review would be highly appreciated.

To your healthy living!

My other books you will love!

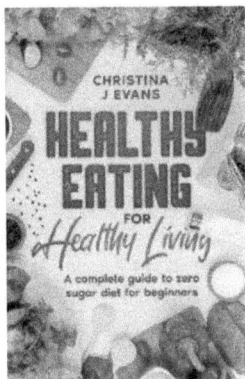

Amazon.com/dp/B09MCXR9T5

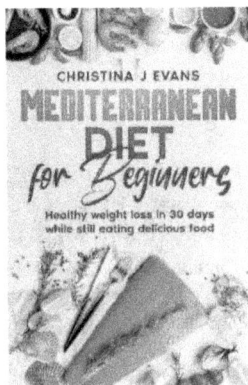

Amazon.com/dp/B09MJ5282Q

Don't forget to grab your GIFT!!!

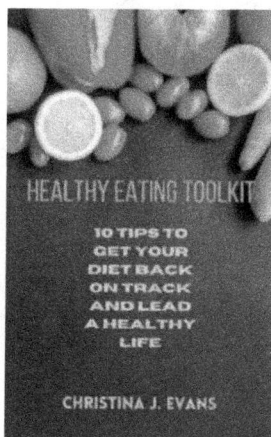

http://christinajevans.com/healthy-eating.pdf

Joining the HL Community

Looking to build your healthy eating lifestyle? If so, then check out the Healthy Living (HL) Community here:

www.facebook.com/groups/1004091000384321/

References

A. (2020a, February 20). *Mediterranean Diet Friendly Chocolate Dipped Strawberries*. Food Wine and Love. https://foodwineandlove.com/mediterranean-diet-friendly-chocolate-dipped-strawberries/

A. (2020b, March 20). *Oil Free Baked Veggie Chips (Paleo, Vegan, Gluten Free)*. The Big Man's World ®. https://thebigmansworld.com/oil-free-baked-veggie-chips-paleo-vegan-gluten-free/#recipe

A. (2020c, March 24). *Mediterranean Diet Ranch Dressing*. Food Wine and Love. https://foodwineandlove.com/mediterranean-diet-ranch-dressing/

A. (2020d, April 20). *Mediterranean Diet Shrimp in Garlic Sauce*. Food Wine and Love. https://foodwineandlove.com/mediterranean-diet-shrimp-in-garlic-sauce/

A. (2020e, October 5). *Chocolate Mousse (no dairy)*. The Mediterranean Movement. https://www.themedimove.com/recipes/diet-recipes/desserts/chocolate-avocado-mousse/

A. (2021a, August 23). *Homemade Trail Mix -*. Fully Mediterranean. https://fullymediterranean.com/recipes/homemade-trail-mix/

Allen, L. (2021, September 8). *Healthy Applesauce Oat Muffins*. Tastes Better From Scratch. https://tastesbetterfromscratch.com/healthy-applesauce-oat-muffins/#recipe

Almond and Brown Rice Pudding. (n.d.). Whole Foods Market. Retrieved October 12, 2021, from https://eu.wholefoodsmarket.com/?destination=www.wholefoodsmarket.com%2Freci pes%2Falmond-brown-rice-pudding

Baked Eggs in Avocado. (2019, April 3). Allrecipes. https://www.allrecipes.com/recipe/240744/paleo-baked-eggs-in-avocado/

Barydakis, K. (2021, September 15). *Tzatziki Sauce: Greek Yogurt, Cucumber, Dill and Garlic*. Mediterranean Living. https://www.mediterraneanliving.com/tzatziki/

Berkowitz, S. F. (2016a, April 29). *Amba pickled mango sauce*. From the Grapevine. https://www.fromthegrapevine.com/israeli-kitchen/recipes/amba-pickled-mango-sauce

Berkowitz, S. F. (2016b, May 2). *Matbucha*. From the Grapevine. https://www.fromthegrapevine.com/israeli-kitchen/recipes/matbucha

Blackberry-Ginger Overnight Bulgur. (2016, August 17). Better Homes & Gardens. https://www.bhg.com/recipe/blackberry-ginger-overnight-bulgur/

Blueberry Lemon Breakfast Quinoa. (2012, December 20). Allrecipes. https://www.allrecipes.com/recipe/230830/blueberry-lemon-breakfast-quinoa/

Bradley, R. B. D. (2021a, September 15). *Balsamic Dill Yogurt Dressing*. Mediterranean Living. https://www.mediterraneanliving.com/balsamic-dill-yogurt-dressing/

Bradley, R. B. D. (2021b, September 15). *Bean Burgers with Garlic and Sage (Vegetarian, Gluten-Free)*. Mediterranean Living. https://www.mediterraneanliving.com/bean-burgers-garlic-sage-vegetarian-gluten-free/

Bradley, R. B. D. (2021c, September 15). *Tangy Italian Salad Dressing*. Mediterranean Living. https://www.mediterraneanliving.com/tangy-italian-salad-dressing/

Bradley, R. B. D. (2021d, October 11). *Mediterranean Fish Stew (30 minute recipe)*. Mediterranean Living. https://www.mediterraneanliving.com/mediterranean-fish-stew-30-minute-recipe/

Bradley, R. B. D. (2021e, October 12). *Cherry Tomato Sauce made in a Mason Jar*. Mediterranean Living. https://www.mediterraneanliving.com/cherry-tomato-sauce-made-in-a-mason-jar/

Cherry-Walnut Overnight Oats. (2018, December 14). EatingWell. https://www.eatingwell.com/recipe/269656/cherry-walnut-overnight-oats/

D. (2020f, January 29). *Italian Salsa Verde Recipe*. Our Salty Kitchen. https://oursaltykitchen.com/italian-salsa-verde/

Delgado, A. M., Almeida, M. D. V., & Parisi, S. (2017). *Chemistry of the Mediterranean diet*. Switzerland: Springer.

DeLeeuw, V. (2021, August 13). *Baked Apple Slices*. Healthy Recipes Blog. https://healthyrecipesblogs.com/baked-apple-slices-recipe/

Devinat, M. (2021a, September 23). *Spinach and Goat Cheese Quiche (France)*. Mediterranean Living. https://www.mediterraneanliving.com/spinach-and-goat-cheese-quiche-france/

Devinat, M. (2021b, September 23). *Tuna Patties Fried in Olive Oil (France)*. Mediterranean Living. https://www.mediterraneanliving.com/tuna-patties-fried-in-olive-oil-france/

Estruch, R., & Ros, E. (2020). *The role of the Mediterranean diet on weight loss and obesity-related diseases*. Reviews in Endocrine and Metabolic Disorders, 21(3), 315-327.

Ezzammoury, M. (2021, September 23). *Moroccan Harira (Lentil, Chickpea and Tomato Soup)*. Mediterranean Living. https://www.mediterraneanliving.com/moroccan-harira-lentil-chickpea-and-tomato-soup/

Feel Good Foodie. (2021, June 5). *Avocado Toast with Egg - 4 Ways*. FeelGoodFoodie. https://feelgoodfoodie.net/recipe/avocado-toast-with-egg-3-ways/#wprm-recipe-container-8175

Fontana, G. (2021a, September 23). *Italian Red Pesto with Sun-Dried Tomatoes and Arugula*. Mediterranean Living. https://www.mediterraneanliving.com/italian-red-pesto-with-sun-dried-tomatoes-and-arugula/

Fontana, G. (2021b, September 23). *Pesto Genovese (Traditional Italian Pesto)*. Mediterranean Living. https://www.mediterraneanliving.com/pesto-genovese-traditional-italian-pesto/

Fontana, G. (2021c, September 23). *Vegetarian Pasta Carbonara*. Mediterranean Living. https://www.mediterraneanliving.com/vegetable-carbonara/

Gib, J. (2006, September 13). *Mediterranean Fruit Salad Recipe - Food.com*. Food. https://www.food.com/recipe/mediterranean-fruit-salad-186006

Greek Turkey Burgers with Spinach, Feta & Tzatziki. (2018, February 6). EatingWell. https://www.eatingwell.com/recipe/262569/greek-turkey-burgers-with-spinach-feta-tzatziki/

Greek-Style Frittata. (2014, September 1). Better Homes & Gardens. https://www.bhg.com/recipe/greek-style-frittata/

H. (2021b, May 23). *Mediterranean Black Bean Salad With Herbs & Feta*. Homemade Mastery. https://www.homemademastery.com/mediterranean-black-bean-salad-with-herbs-feta/

HasanzadeNemati, S. (2021, May 3). *Mediterranean Baked Dijon Salmon Recipe [Video]*. Unicorns in the Kitchen. https://www.unicornsinthekitchen.com/mediterranean-baked-dijon-salmon-recipe-video/#recipe/

Hasselback Caprese Chicken. (2017, November 16). EatingWell. https://www.eatingwell.com/recipe/261639/hasselback-caprese-chicken/

Hesser, A. (2019, August 20). *Olive Oil Gelato*. Food52. https://food52.com/recipes/10866-olive-oil-gelato

K. (2019a, January 31). *Mediterranean Roasted Chickpeas Recipe*. A Simple Pantry. https://asimplepantry.com/roasted-chickpeas-recipe/

K. (2020g, May 22). *Best Tahini Sauce*. Cookie and Kate. https://cookieandkate.com/best-tahini-sauce-recipe/

Kale Chips. (n.d.). Carb Manager. Retrieved October 12, 2021, from https://www.carbmanager.com/recipe-detail/ug:9977456c-74f2-45e2-24e2-3959d917652b/keto-mediterranean-kale-chips

L. (2021c, April 2). *Easy Homemade Flatbread Crackers*. Pinch of Yum. https://pinchofyum.com/easy-homemade-flatbread-crackers

LeBlanc, G. (2021, September 15). *Baked Cod with Sun-Dried Tomatoes and Olives*. Mediterranean Living. https://www.mediterraneanliving.com/baked-cod-sun-dried-tomatoes-olives/

M. (2017, June 28). *Strawberry popsicles*. Tasty Mediterraneo. https://www.tastymediterraneo.com/strawberry-popsicles/

M. (2020h, March 2). *Mediterranean style guacamole*. Tasty Mediterraneo. https://www.tastymediterraneo.com/mediterranean-style-guacamole/

Martínez-González, M. Á., De la Fuente-Arrillaga, C., Nunez-Cordoba, J. M., Basterra-Gortari, F. J., Beunza, J. J., Vazquez, Z., ... & Bes-Rastrollo, M. (2008). *Adherence to Mediterranean diet and risk of developing diabetes: prospective cohort study*. Bmj, 336(7657), 1348-1351.

Martínez-González, M. Á., Hershey, M. S., Zazpe, I., & Trichopoulou, A. (2017). *Transferability of the Mediterranean diet to non-Mediterranean countries. What is and what is not the Mediterranean diet*. Nutrients, 9(11), 1226.

McDowell, B. (2021, March 3). *Chia Pomegranate Smoothie*. The Domestic Dietitian. https://thedomesticdietitian.com/chia-pomegranate-smoothie/

Mediterranean Cauliflower Pizza. (2016, June 3). EatingWell. https://www.eatingwell.com/recipe/250891/mediterranean-cauliflower-pizza/

Mediterranean Chickpea Quinoa Bowl. (2017, May 11). EatingWell. https://www.eatingwell.com/recipe/258195/mediterranean-chickpea-quinoa-bowl/

Mediterranean Grilled Sea Bass. (2021, April 30). Good Housekeeping. https://www.goodhousekeeping.com/food-recipes/a6026/mediterranean-grilled-sea-bass-2200/

Mediterranean Sweet and Sour Chicken. (2019, June 5). Good Housekeeping. https://www.goodhousekeeping.com/food-recipes/a5393/mediterranean-sweet-sour-chicken-1815/

Mindbody green. (2018, January 10). *Coconut, Tahini, and Cashew Bars*. https://www.mindbodygreen.com/articles/blood-sugar-balancing-tahini-dessert

Morris, N. A. D. (2021, September 15). *Yogurt Tahini Dip and Dressing*. Mediterranean Living. https://www.mediterraneanliving.com/yogurt-tahini-dip-and-dressing/

Murray, T., & Murray, T. (2021, June 7). *Shakshuka*. Good Housekeeping. https://www.goodhousekeeping.com/food-recipes/a34908201/easy-shakshuka-recipe/

One-Pot Greek Pasta. (2018, February 28). EatingWell. https://www.eatingwell.com/recipe/262954/one-pot-greek-pasta/

P. (2021d, August 23). *Peach Soup -*. Fully Mediterranean. https://fullymediterranean.com/recipes/peach-soup/

Paoli, A., Bianco, A., Grimaldi, K. A., Lodi, A., & Bosco, G. (2013). *Long term successful weight loss with a combination biphasic ketogenic mediterranean diet and mediterranean diet maintenance protocol*. Nutrients, 5(12), 5205-5217.

Pineapple Green Smoothie. (2016, June 3). EatingWell. https://www.eatingwell.com/recipe/251038/pineapple-green-smoothie/

Quinoa & Chia Oatmeal Mix. (2016, October 12). EatingWell. https://www.eatingwell.com/recipe/255762/quinoa-chia-oatmeal-mix/

Quinoa Avocado Salad. (2018, April 19). EatingWell.
https://www.eatingwell.com/recipe/264061/quinoa-avocado-salad/
Rinaldi de Alvarenga, J. F., Quifer-Rada, P., Westrin, V., Hurtado-Barroso, S., Torrado-
Prat, X., & Lamuela-Raventós, R. M. (2019*). Mediterranean sofrito home-cooking
technique enhances polyphenol content in tomato sauce.* Journal of the Science of
Food and Agriculture, 99(14), 6535-6545.
S. (2019b, December 30). *Tabouli Salad Recipe (Tabbouleh).* The Mediterranean Dish.
https://www.themediterraneandish.com/tabouli-salad/
S. (2020i, April 17). *Crispy Homemade Fish Sticks.* The Mediterranean Dish.
https://www.themediterraneandish.com/homemade-fish-sticks/
S. (2020j, May 17). *Easy Baba Ganoush Recipe.* The Mediterranean Dish.
https://www.themediterraneandish.com/baba-ganoush-recipe/
S. (2020k, June 10). *Healthy Tomato, Basil, and Chickpea Salad - Vegan and Gluten-
Free.* Beauty Bites. https://www.beautybites.org/healthy-tomatoes-basil-chickpea-
salad-vegan-gluten-free/
S. (2020l, August 17). *Easy Roasted Tomato Basil Soup (Vegan, GF).* The
Mediterranean Dish. https://www.themediterraneandish.com/vegan-roasted-tomato-
basil-soup/
S. (2020m, December 7). *Easy Greek Red Lentil Soup.* The Mediterranean Dish.
https://www.themediterraneandish.com/red-lentil-soup-recipe/
S. (2020n, December 16). *Maple Vanilla Baked Pears.* Sally's Baking Addiction.
https://sallysbakingaddiction.com/simple-maple-vanilla-baked-pears/
S. (2021e, January 6). *Creamy Tahini Date Banana Shake.* The Mediterranean Dish.
https://www.themediterraneandish.com/tahini-date-banana-shake/
S. (2021f, February 1). *Baked Zucchini with Parmesan and Thyme.* The Mediterranean
Dish. https://www.themediterraneandish.com/easy-baked-zucchini/
S. (2021g, March 20). *Simple Italian Minestrone Soup.* The Mediterranean Dish.
https://www.themediterraneandish.com/simple-italian-minestrone-soup/
S. (2021h, September 3). *Mediterranean Grilled Chicken Kabobs.* The Mediterranean
Dish. https://www.themediterraneandish.com/mediterranean-grilled-chicken-kabobs-
tahini-sauce/
Sahyoun, N. R., & Sankavaram, K. (2016). *Historical origins of the Mediterranean
diet, regional dietary profiles, and the development of the dietary guidelines.* In
Mediterranean Diet (pp. 43-56). Humana Press, Cham.
Segrave-Daly, D. (2020, June 19). *Grilled Watermelon Salad: Grilled Fruit Recipe
Roundup.* Teaspoon of Spice | Serena Ball MS, RD, & Deanna Segrave-Daly, RD.
https://teaspoonofspice.com/grilled-watermelon-salad-grilled-fruit-recipes/
Stuffed Eggplant. (2016, June 3). EatingWell.
https://www.eatingwell.com/recipe/253027/stuffed-eggplant/

Taste of Home Editors. (2021, September 25). *Mediterranean Shrimp Linguine*. Taste of Home. https://www.tasteofhome.com/recipes/mediterranean-shrimp-linguine/

Tercero, S. (2021, September 28). *Muhammara (Roasted Red Pepper and Walnut Dip)*. Mediterranean Living. https://www.mediterraneanliving.com/muhammara-roasted-red-pepper-and-walnut-dip/

Trichopoulou, A., & Vasilopoulou, E. (2000). *Mediterranean diet and longevity*. British Journal of Nutrition, 84(S2), S205-S209.

Watermelon and Mint Granita. (2017, August 10). The Best of Bridge. https://www.bestofbridge.com/watermelon-and-mint-granita/

Willett, W. C., Sacks, F., Trichopoulou, A., Drescher, G., Ferro-Luzzi, A., Helsing, E., & Trichopoulos, D. (1995). *Mediterranean diet pyramid: a cultural model for healthy eating*. The American journal of clinical nutrition, 61(6), 1402S-1406S.

Urquiaga, I., Echeverria, G., Dussaillant, C., & Rigotti, A. (2017). *Origin, components, and mechanisms of action of the Mediterranean diet*. Revista medica de Chile, 145(1), 85-95.

Yogurt with Blueberries & Honey. (2017, November 16). EatingWell. https://www.eatingwell.com/recipe/261617/yogurt-with-blueberries-honey/

Zikos, B. B. G. (2021, September 15). *Lebanese Hummus*. Mediterranean Living. https://www.mediterraneanliving.com/lebanese-hummus/

Zikos, G. (2021a, September 15). *Sheet Pan Baked Eggplant Parmesan*. Mediterranean Living. https://www.mediterraneanliving.com/sheet-pan-baked-eggplant-parmesan/

Zikos, G. (2021b, October 8). *Sheet Pan Chicken Thighs with Peppers and Onions*. Mediterranean Living. https://www.mediterraneanliving.com/sheet-pan-chicken-thighs-with-peppers-and-onions/

Zucchini with Egg. (2020, June 19). Allrecipes. https://www.allrecipes.com/recipe/242245/zucchini-with-egg/

Dump and Bake Chicken Fajita Bake With Quinoa - The .... https://www.theseasonedmom.com/dump-bake-chicken-fajita-quinoa/

www.ingramcontent.com/pod-product-compliance
Lightning Source LLC
Chambersburg PA
CBHW020248030426
42336CB00010B/672